Stroke in childhood

Clinical guidelines for diagnosis, management and rehabilitation

Prepared by the Paediatric Stroke Working Group

November 2004

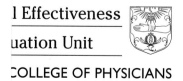

l Effectiveness
uation Unit

COLLEGE OF PHYSICIANS

The Clinical Effectiveness and Evaluation Unit

The Clinical Effectiveness and Evaluation Unit (CEEU) of the Royal College of Physicians has expertise in the develoment of evidence-based guidelines and the organising and reporting of multicentre comparative performance data. The work programme is collaborative and multiprofessional, involving the relevant specialist societies and patient groups, the National Institute for Clinical Excellence (NICE) and the Healthcare Commission. The CEEU is self-financing with funding from national health service bodies, the Royal College of Physicians, charities and other organisations.

Acknowledgement

The development of these guidelines was supported by funding from a variety of sources including: The Stroke Association, Different Strokes, Boehringer Ingelheim, Merck Sharp & Dohme, and Sanofi-Synthelabo & Bristol-Myers Squibb.

The Royal College of Physicians is also pleased to acknowledge a grant from The Haymills Charitable Trust towards the cost of designing and printing the guidelines.

Front cover

Design by Merriton Sharp, London.

The cover photograph, of a young boy who suffered a stroke at 15 months but who has made an almost complete recovery, is used by kind permission of Derek and Jane Walker and Different Strokes.

Different Strokes, 9 Canon Harnett Court, Wolverton Mill, Milton Keynes MK12 5NF. Tel: 0845 130 71 72; E-mail: info@differentstrokes.co.uk; Website: www.differentstrokes.co.uk.

Website addresses

Every effort has been made to ensure that the website addresses in this document are valid at the time of going to press. However, readers should be aware that they may be subject to change over time.

Royal College of Physicians of London
11 St Andrews Place, London NW1 4LE

Registered Charity No 210508

Copyright © 2004 Royal College of Physicians of London

ISBN 1 86016 236 3

Text design by the Publications Unit of the Royal College of Physicians
Typeset by Dan-Set Graphics, Telford, Shropshire
Printed in Great Britain by The Lavenham Press Ltd, Suffolk

The Paediatric Stroke Working Group

Vijeya Ganesan (Chair)
Senior Lecturer in Paediatric Neurology, Institute of Child Health, University College London

Kling Chong
Consultant Neuroradiologist, Great Ormond Street Hospital for Children NHS Trust

Jane Evans
Consultant Paediatric Haematologist, University College London Hospital

Anne Gordon
Research Occupational Therapist, Institute of Child Health, University College London

Dianne Gumley
Consultant Clinical Psychologist, Great Ormond Street Hospital for Children NHS Trust

Penny Irwin
Stroke Programme Co-ordinator, Royal College of Physicians, London

Fenella Kirkham
Reader in Paediatric Neurology, Institute of Child Health, University College London

Janet Lees
Consultant Speech and Language Therapist and Honorary Lecturer, Department of Human Communication Sciences, University of Sheffield, and Honorary Research Fellow, Neurosciences Unit, Institute of Child Health, University College London

Donal O'Kelly
Different Strokes

Terry Pountney
Senior Physiotherapist, Chailey Heritage School, East Sussex

Eoin Redahan
The Stroke Association

Susan Rideout
Clinical Specialist Paediatric Neurology, Physiotherapy Department, Birmingham Children's Hospital

Dominic Thompson
Consultant Neurosurgeon, Great Ormond Street Hospital for Children NHS Trust

Beth Ward
Clinical Nurse Specialist, Great Ormond Street Hospital for Children

Sue Wayne
The Stroke Association

Andrew Williams
Consultant Community Paediatrician, Northampton General Hospital

Keith Wood
Different Strokes

Sickle cell subgroup

Kofi Anie
Consultant Clinical Psychologist, Brent Sickle Cell & Thalassaemia Centre

Lola Oni
Nurse Director/Lecturer, Brent Sickle Cell & Thalassaemia Centre

Contents

Foreword

Stroke, in both adults and children, used to be something that happened but which medicine could do, or chose to do, little about. Over the last decade there has been a revolution in stroke care for adults, with the advent of specialist stroke units and evolving treatments. Publication of the first edition of the *National clinical guidelines for stroke* in 2000 and the National Sentinel Audit of Stroke stimulated local units to consider the quality of the care they were delivering and put improvements in place. Rehabilitative care after stroke for adults is now considered the norm, and the collaboration between physicians, nurses, therapists and patients in these projects has led to true multidisciplinary working – much to the benefit of patients.

Similar improvements, however, have not been seen in the treatment of childhood stroke which, although less common than adult stroke, is still a serious problem and one which anecdotal evidence suggests is prone to an even more variable quality of care. Thus, when the national guidelines were being revised by the Intercollegiate Stroke Working Party, a subgroup was formed to consider the paediatric aspects of stroke care. During development it became clear that little evidence existed for many areas. The gaps were filled using the expertise of the group and the views of patients, parents and carers, but it is clear that there is a need for more formal research.

This guideline is aimed at healthcare staff in all parts of the NHS and related services, but much of it may also be of value to patients, parents and families. It is hoped that it will help childhood stroke services to emulate the improvement that has occurred, and is continuing to occur, in the care of adults, bringing a consistency and a knowledge of best practice to an area marked until now by dislocated care and uncertain standards.

To the casual reader wondering if this is important – I would urge you to begin by glancing at the italicised quotes from participants in the child and carer workshop which are scattered through the document. They plainly show how much more should and can be done to ensure good acute management, rehabilitation and secondary prevention, and to help these young people and their parents and families adjust to and cope with the effects of their stroke. Children have a lifetime ahead of them – any benefits from improved care will also last a lifetime.

November 2004

Professor Mike Pearson
Director, Clinical Effectiveness and Evaluation Unit,
Royal College of Physicians

The child and family perspective

As part of the guideline development process a workshop was held for children affected by stroke and their families. It gave a sense of the issues children and families felt to be important. We particularly focused on these issues in developing the guidelines, and they are outlined here.

The child is part of a family and, therefore, any childhood illness will have effects on both the immediate and extended family. The diagnosis of stroke is an unexpected one in a child, which compounds the shock experienced by families at the time of diagnosis.

The lack of information for families of children affected by stroke was a strong theme in the workshop. Information on what has happened and what to expect could empower families to ensure that the immediate and long-term needs of their child can be met. Information for parents, carers and children should be designed to meet their specific needs. The same information pack is unlikely to be appropriate in all cases but the information leaflet provided with this document may form a useful starting point. It is important that the questions asked by parents, carers, and children are answered. The communication of information to children is often particularly neglected.

Parents and carers of children affected by stroke welcome support from those who have had similar experiences – they appreciate someone to talk to about what has happened and to help them look at the future. Children also welcome meetings with those in their own age group affected by stroke. Both parents and children explained that the diagnosis of stroke is traumatic and that they need help in adjusting. It is important for families to see that life goes on. At the end of this document there is a list of useful organisations, including support groups, which may be able to provide information and support.

Families commented on significant gaps in communication between the various professional teams involved in the care of a child affected by stroke, and, as discussed above, between professionals and the family. This is an area which is extensively addressed in the guidelines.

There are significant problems in accessing therapy following childhood stroke in some areas. It is important that there is a coherent plan for rehabilitation which takes into account all of the child's needs and which can be met within local resources. Gaps in service provision should be highlighted and brought to the attention of service planners.

Introduction

1 Introduction

1.1 Background

Childhood stroke is a neglected area, with both professionals and the general public lacking awareness of the problem and its potential consequences. Stroke affects several hundred children in the UK each year and is one of the top ten causes of childhood death (Fullerton *et al* 2002). Many children who have a stroke have another medical condition (such as a cardiac disorder or sickle cell disease) and, therefore, are already vulnerable to adverse neurodevelopmental effects (Lanthier *et al* 2000, Ganesan *et al* 2003). The prevalence of sickle cell disease varies widely within the United Kingdom. However, it is noteworthy that at least 10% of these children and young people will have a stroke during childhood. The burden of childhood stroke on the health services is, numerically, smaller than stroke in the elderly. However, the long-lasting physical, emotional and social effects of stroke on an individual near the beginning of their life affect not only the individual themselves, but also their family and society as a whole.

Many professional agencies can be involved in helping the affected child fulfil their potential and in providing support and advice to the family. These agencies may change in the course of the child's life and it is important that they are all aware of the consequences of childhood stroke, and that their efforts are co-ordinated. The child's cognitive, social and emotional needs are in constant evolution and the functional impact of childhood stroke may, as a consequence, vary over time.

We have taken a child-centred approach to formulating these guidelines, working in partnership with children, families and support groups, specifically seeking the views of children and families, and centring the guidelines on issues raised by them. Throughout this document use of the term 'parents' is intended to encompass the child's parents and any other carers.

The large number of consensus statements and good practice points in these guidelines emphasise that research in the field of childhood stroke is urgently needed to provide definitive answers to many of the issues raised. There is an acknowledged need for multicentre collaboration in such research to enable the design of studies with sufficient power to produce definitive results. The networks necessary for this are beginning to be established and may lead to work which could provide a firmer evidence base for the care of children affected by stroke.

Participant in paediatric stroke workshop: I am not a stroke, I have had one.

3

1.2 Scope of the guidelines

These guidelines will primarily address the diagnosis, investigation and management of acute arterial ischaemic stroke in children beyond the neonatal period (aged one month to 18 years at time of presentation), including acute presentation and management, rehabilitation and longer-term care. Many of the issues covered here, in particular those relating to rehabilitation, will also be relevant to children with other causes of stroke (for example cerebral venous infarction, neonatal stroke or intracranial haemorrhage).

1.3 Purpose of the guidelines

These guidelines are aimed at professionals working in primary care, secondary level acute and community paediatrics, tertiary level paediatric neurology and neurodisability, education, and social services. The aim of the guidelines is to provide evidence-based recommendations for clinicians.

1.4 Methodology

These guidelines were formulated in accordance with the principles specified by the Appraisal of Guidelines Research and Evaluation (AGREE) collaboration (**www.agreecollaboration.org**)

Following the publication of the National Clinical Guidelines for Stroke in 2000 (Intercollegiate Working Party for Stroke 2000) – referred to hereafter, along with the second edition (Intercollegiate Stroke Working Party 2004), as the 'adult guidelines' – several parties approached the Royal College of Physicians inquiring about guidelines for childhood stroke. The British Paediatric Neurology Association instigated a working party to formulate guidelines. This work was done in collaboration with the Clinical Effectiveness and Evaluation Unit of the Royal College of Physicians. Potential members were identified through their recognised record of clinical and research activity in the field of paediatric stroke and also through their professional organisations. Representation was sought across a broad range of disciplines and two patient organisations (the Stroke Association and Different Strokes). The members of the working party are listed at the front of this book. Conflicts of interest were declared and monitored (and full statements held on file).

The working party began by constructing a list of headings using the existing adult stroke guidelines (Intercollegiate Working Party for Stroke 2000) as a reference. We also considered specific additional issues relevant to children (for example, return to school). For each area, the group decided on a list of specific questions that would be considered. Searches were done using key words relevant to these questions of available computerised databases from 1966 onwards: Medline, AMED, CINAHL and Embase. In addition, the Cochrane Collaboration database was searched and other national guidelines and publications were reviewed. Members of the working party brought their own expertise and knowledge of the literature, as well as information from their organisations and professional bodies.

Topics were divided and allocated to individual members for evaluation according to their expertise. These individuals had responsibility for appraising the evidence and drafting the recommendations. The Scottish Intercollegiate Guidelines Network (SIGN 50) guidelines appraisal checklists were used to assess the quality of published articles (**www.sign.ac.uk/ guidelines**). Guidelines were written on the basis of the available evidence with grading of the strength of the recommendation and explanatory statements where necessary. All recommendations were then presented to the working party as a whole for discussion and agreement.

Selection of articles for inclusion was based on the following principles. Where evidence specifically relating to childhood stroke was available, this alone was used. However, such literature is extremely limited and, therefore, research from other paediatric neurological conditions was evaluated where these conditions were felt to be relevant to the issues being considered. If a recommendation was based on extrapolation from research in a different population to that covered by the guideline, the grade of recommendation was reduced by one level.

Where evidence from meta-analyses or randomised controlled trials (RCTs) was available, this was used. Where there was limited or no evidence from RCTs, then evidence from observational group studies or small-group studies was used. In general, evidence from single-case studies was not used, primarily because it is difficult to draw general conclusions from them. Where there was no evidence base to support guidelines in areas which were highly relevant to clinical practice, consensus statements from this working party, other working parties and professional bodies were used. Many recommendations are in line with those in the developing National Service Framework for Children (**www.dh.gov.uk/ PolicyAndGuidance/HealthAndSocialCareTopics/ChildrenServices/fs/en**).

The strength of evidence and recommendations were graded using the scheme proposed by SIGN 50 and summarised in tables 1.1 and 1.2, overleaf. The 'Evidence' sections following guidelines give an indication of the nature and extent of the supporting evidence, together with key references. Lastly, for each topic, there is an evidence table or group of evidence tables giving further details of the main studies.

Children affected by stroke and their parents were invited to attend a structured workshop in order to identify areas they thought should be addressed within the guidelines. The findings were used to identify key themes, which were subsequently incorporated into the issues addressed by the guidelines.

All the guidelines have been peer reviewed by external reviewers, a group which included a range of stakeholders (see Appendix 1).

Table 1.1 Guideline strength: levels of evidence

Level of evidence	Type of evidence
1++	High quality meta-analyses, systematic reviews of RCTs, or RCTs with a very low risk of bias
1+	Well-conducted meta-analyses, systematic reviews of RCTs, or RCTs with a low risk of bias
1–	Meta-analyses, systematic reviews of RCTs, or RCTs with a high risk of bias
2++	High quality systematic reviews of case control or cohort studies; high quality case control or cohort studies with a very low risk of confounding, bias or chance and a high probability that the relationship is causal
2+	Well-conducted case control or cohort studies with a low risk of confounding, bias or chance and a moderate probability that the relationship is causal
2–	Case control or cohort studies with a high risk of confounding, bias or chance and a significant risk that the relationship is not causal
3	Non-analytic studies, eg case reports, case series
4	Expert opinion

Table 1.2 Guideline strength: grades of recommendation

Grade of recommendation	Evidence
A	At least one meta-analysis, systematic review or RCT rated as 1++, and directly applicable to the target population; or, a systematic review of RCTs or a body of evidence consisting principally of studies rated as 1+, directly applicable to the target population and demonstrating overall consistency of results
B	A body of evidence including studies rated as 2++, directly applicable to the target population, and demonstrating overall consistency of results; or, extrapolated evidence from studies rated as 1++ or 1+
C	A body of evidence including studies rated as 2+, directly applicable to the target population and demonstrating overall consistency of results; or extrapolated evidence from studies rated as 2++
D	Evidence level 3 or 4; or, extrapolated evidence from studies rated as 2+
✓	A tick after a guideline represents a 'good practice point' – the recommended best practice based on the clinical experience of the guideline development group

1.5 Context and use

These guidelines are intended to inform clinical decisions rather than to be rigidly applied.

2 Terminology and theoretical framework

A factor interfering with delivery of good stroke care for children is the lack of a widely accepted framework of care and universal vocabulary and terminology. Health professionals have widely varying experiences of childhood stroke, but the problem is exacerbated by the variation in expertise and preferences for intervention in the absence of an accepted framework. The revised World Health Organization (WHO) classification (International Classification of Functioning, Disability and Health (ICF)) is intended to include all aspects of the health of an individual throughout life. This is designed to replace the former ICIDH (International Classification of Impairments, Disabilities and Handicap), which was widely accepted and used in describing health.

2.1 The International Classification of Functioning, Disability and Health

ICF classifies health and health-related states. The unit of classification is 'categories' within health and health-related domains. It is important to note, therefore, that in the ICF persons are not the units of classification; that is, ICF does not classify people, but describes the situation of each person within an array of health or health-related domains. Moreover, the description is always within the context of environmental and personal factors. This interaction can be viewed as a *process* or a *result* depending on the user. For an example of how the ICF might be used in practice, see Appendix 3.

Overview of ICF components

In the context of health:

▶ **body functions** are the physiological functions of body systems (including psychological functions)

▶ **body structures** are anatomical parts of the body such as organs, limbs and their components

▶ **impairments** are problems in body function or structure such as a significant deviation or loss

▶ **activity** is the execution of a task or action by an individual

▶ **participation** is involvement in a life situation

▶ **activity limitations** are difficulties an individual may have in executing activities

▶ **participation restrictions** are problems an individual may experience in involvement in life situations

---

► **environmental factors** make up the physical, social and attitudinal environment in which people live and conduct their lives.

An overview of these concepts is given [in the table below]. As the table indicates:

► ICF has two *parts*, each with two *components:*

Part 1. Functioning and Disability

(a) Body Functions and Structures

(b) Activities and Participation

Part 2. Contextual Factors

(a) Environmental Factors

(b) Personal Factors

► Each component can be expressed in both *positive* and *negative* terms...

An overview of ICF

	Part 1: Functioning and Disability		Part 2: Contextual Factors	
Components	Body Functions and Structures	Activities and Participation	Environmental Factors	Personal Factors
Domains	Body functions Body sructures	Life Areas (tasks, actions)	External influences on functioning and disability	Internal influences on functioning and disability
Constructs	Change in body functions (physiological) Change in body structures (anatomical)	Capacity Executing tasks in a standard environment Performance Executing tasks in the current environment	Facilitating or hindering impact of features of the physical, social and attitudinal world	Impact of attributes of the person
Positive Aspect	Functional and structural integrity	Activities Participation	Facilitators	not applicable
	Functioning			
Negative Aspect	Impairment	Activity limitation Participation restriction	Barriers / hindrances	not applicable
	Disability			

Source: World Health Organization (2001) *ICF: International Classification of Functioning Disability and Health.* WHO: Geneva. Available at: **www3.who.int/icf/icftemplate.cfm**

Guidelines

1 Each team should use a consistent framework and terminology in providing care to the child affected by stroke ☑

2 It is recommended that the World Health Organization's International Classification of Functioning (ICF) terminology is used ☑

Evidence

1 & 2 Working party consensus

The guidelines

3 Service organisation

Children affected by stroke make use of all levels of health, education and social services in the United Kingdom. From a medical perspective the patient journey can be considered in terms of acute medical care, and both acute and longer-term rehabilitation. Rehabilitation should be integrated with the child's educational, social and emotional needs.

In contrast to adult stroke, where the model is to develop specialist stroke services, the relative rarity of childhood stroke means that existing primary, secondary and tertiary systems of child health will – appropriately – be involved. These services and their potential roles are outlined in Table 3.1, overleaf. Services for the rehabilitation and longer-term needs of children with any acquired brain injury, including stroke, are relatively underdeveloped in the United Kingdom; in fact, their care challenges services and processes in both health and education, which are typically built around the needs of children with much more stable, slowly changing requirements (eg those with cerebral palsy). Although the development of more accurately targeted services is being proposed, the following section will describe the potential roles, and involvement in the management of children affected by stroke, of services as they are currently structured. The wide variation in the nature and potential severity of the long-term effects of stroke means that it is difficult to propose a single approach which would be suitable for all children, and the applicability of each recommendation to the specific child and family should be considered.

It is our view that all children affected by acute stroke should be referred to a consultant paediatric neurologist. However, it may not always be appropriate for the child to be transferred to an acute paediatric neurology unit. If this is the case, the child's management should be discussed with the tertiary level paediatric neurology service. At present many, but not all, tertiary paediatric neurology units have multidisciplinary teams with expertise in the evaluation of children with acquired neurological problems. However in other tertiary centres, and many secondary centres, formal acute-based teams do not exist and are convened on an *ad hoc* basis. Where specialist expertise is not available locally professionals are encouraged to liaise with, and obtain advice from, colleagues in specialist centres. The needs of the child must remain central to the consideration of which professionals to involve.

The lack of structured paediatric rehabilitation services could be attributed to i) a lack of research regarding long-term outcomes of acquired brain injury in childhood, ii) a misplaced optimism regarding the plasticity of the child's brain and the potential for recovery, iii) a lack of appreciation of the developmental context, and the fact that effects not apparent immediately may emerge with time, iv) a lack of recognition of the 'invisible' consequences of brain injury (for example, cognitive or emotional effects). These factors all need to be taken into account when considering the services available to children affected by stroke. The

Table 3.1 Composition of current paediatric services in the United Kingdom and potential roles in the care of children affected by stroke

Service	Professionals	Roles
Tertiary care services		
Specialist children's hospital	– Paediatric neurologist – Nursing staff – Allied health professionals (occupational therapist, physiotherapist, speech and language therapist) – Clinical psychologist – Social worker – Other tertiary level paediatric specialists	– Establish diagnosis – Acute medical (or surgical) treatment – Early disability assessment and treatment during inpatient period – Liaison with secondary acute and community services (including provision of advice and support to secondary services after discharge)
Specialist children's rehabilitation unit	– Paediatrician with neurodisability or rehabilitation training – Nursing staff – Allied health professionals – Educational psychologist – Teacher – Child and adolescent mental health professionals	– Assessment of impairment and disability – Rehabilitation – Plan for transition to community services – Liaison with secondary acute and community services (including provision of advice and support to secondary services after discharge)
Secondary care services		
Acute paediatrics	– Consultant paediatrician – Nursing staff – Allied health professionals – Social worker – Teacher	– Establish diagnosis – Acute medical treatment – Early disability assessment and treatment during inpatient period – May take on longer-term rehabilitation depending on availability of local services – Liaison with tertiary hospital and community services
Community child health	Child development service usually includes (*Standards for child development services* (RCPCH 1999)): – Consultant paediatrician – Community nurse – Allied health professionals – Clinical psychologist – Social worker – Portage worker – Teacher – Child psychiatrist – Educational psychologist	– Assessment of impairments and disabilities – Set up and deliver long-term package of care – Liaison with educational and social services, secondary and tertiary hospital paediatric services
Primary care services		
General practice	– General practitioner – Health visitor – Community nurse	– Ongoing developmental surveillance – Management of general medical issues – Liaison with secondary and tertiary care services as required

proposed national working group to develop a paediatric rehabilitation policy would be highly relevant to children affected by stroke. At present there are only 50 specialist paediatric rehabilitation beds in the UK. This means that the rehabilitation of the majority of children affected by stroke will take place either in the community or on general paediatric wards.

Multidisciplinary assessment and co-ordination, and the provision of long-term care, are usually undertaken by community child health services, most often by the child development service. It is also at this level that ongoing liaison between health, social and education services should occur. In many areas there will be a specific team, usually based in a child development centre, responsible for children aged five and under with disabilities (*Standards for child development services* (RCPCH 1999)). The community child health service, alongside professionals in the education services, will also be involved in the management of school age children. It is important that services are not duplicated and that all those involved are clear on who is taking the lead.

Primary care services are usually involved in general health issues, and the child's general practitioner should be routinely and regularly informed by tertiary and secondary services of a child's health and the services they are using. The health visitor may play an important co-ordinating role within the multidisciplinary team.

Effective multi- and inter-agency working is essential to ensure comprehensive care in the rehabilitation of children with acquired brain injury. This is also emphasised in several documents, for example *Together from the start* (DfES 2002), and the *Standards for child development services* (RCPCH 1999). Developments in information sharing resources, such as the forthcoming Integrated Children's System (DfES) should facilitate multi- and interagency working.

The aim of team-working is to provide a smooth, coordinated and integrated service for children and their families. A 'team' is defined as a group of people working towards a single goal or set of goals, but it is important that this is an interactive effort. The aim of the multidisciplinary team is to provide a holistic perspective of the child and family in planning or providing interventions, and to stop any duplication of questions, assessments or services.

The model of having a key worker for the child and family is controversial and has not been researched in this group of children. However, documents relating to the management of children with disability (for example *Together from the start* (DfES 2002) and *Standards for child development services* (RCPCH 1999)) as well as the recent green paper, *Every child matters* (DH 2003b), advocate such a model. Given the complex and evolving nature of the potential consequences of childhood stroke and the multitude of agencies which could be involved, we feel that a key worker is likely to increase the likelihood of delivering a co-ordinated care package. A key worker is defined as a person who 'works in partnership with the family, with the function of co-ordinating service provision and serving as a point of reference for the family' (*Together from the start*, DfES 2002). A further critical aspect of this role is that the key worker takes responsibility for ensuring delivery of the package of care. Any professional could take on the role of key worker, but it is likely to be most appropriate that this is a member of the secondary level team. Additional factors which should influence the choice of the key worker are the preference of the child and family and the key worker's competencies. The family should be given clear information about the identity and role of their key worker.

Guidelines

1 All children with acute stroke should be referred to, or have their management discussed with, a consultant paediatric neurologist ✓

2 Where specialist expertise is not available locally, professionals from all disciplines are encouraged to liaise with, and obtain advice from, colleagues in specialist centres regarding the acute assessment and management of the child affected by stroke ✓

3 Care should be provided in an environment that is appropriate for the child's age and developmental level (**D**)

4 The medical, social, emotional and educational needs of the child affected by stroke should be considered early and systematically assessed in a co-ordinated manner when planning their subsequent care (**D**)

5 All members of the healthcare team should work together with the child and family, using an agreed therapeutic approach (**D**)

6 The longer-term management of the child affected by stroke should be co-ordinated by a consultant paediatrician ✓

7 A multidisciplinary team with expertise in the care of children with neurological conditions should be involved in the management of the child affected by stroke. Whilst this may initially be at tertiary level, it is essential that the relevant secondary level child development service is involved from an early stage ✓

8 A key worker should be appointed to co-ordinate the package of care, ensure its delivery and to act as a central point of contact for the family (**D**). The key worker and their role should be explained to the family

Evidence

1 Consensus of working party

2 Consensus of working party

3 Recommendation 18 of *Learning from Bristol: the report of the public inquiry into children's heart surgery at the Bristol Royal infirmary 1984–1995* (**www.bristol-inquiry.org.uk**); Children's National Service Framework (**www.dh. gov.uk**) (**4**)

4 *Together from the start* (DfES 2002) (**4**); *Standards for child development services* (RCPCH 1999) (**4**)

5 *Standards for child development services* (RCPCH 1999) (**4**)

6 Consensus of working party

7 Consensus of working party

8 *Together from the start* (DfES 2002) (**4**); *Standards for child development services* (RCPCH 1999) (**4**)

4 Children and their families

4.1 Consent

Children, whatever their age, have a right to be consulted and informed about any proposed treatment. The UN Convention on Children's Rights recognises the right of children to make informed decisions. Information (either verbal or written) needs to be accessible to children. Their dignity, self-respect, and rights to self-determination and non-interference should be preserved (**www.unicef.org/crc/crc.htm**).

The Children Act 1989 and European Association for Children in Hospital charter (**www.each-for-sick-children.org/charter.htm**) require that children and parents participate in decision-making. Children's feelings and wishes should be sought and taken into account, and any reasons for not following them should be explained. Religious persuasion, racial origin, culture and language should also be considered. Children should be protected from unnecessary treatment and interference. The Gillick Judgement (*Gillick v West Norfolk Health Authority* 1985) requires that consent be given by a child if they have 'sufficient understanding and intelligence to enable understanding fully what is proposed, even if under the age of consent'.

4.2 Families and carers

The child and family perspective

'*I wanted to know… if I could use my hand normally, how long it would take to heal*' (participant in paediatric stroke workshop).

Parents of affected children had experienced '*not being told what is going on*' and '*being kept in the dark*'. Parents and carers also reported feelings of helplessness, distress and guilt from witnessing their children's pain and fear and being unable to help them: '*I felt helpless, I couldn't do anything for her*', '*I rushed … to the hospital, all I could hear was my niece screaming … I cried, saying to myself she's only 15 years old*', '*Seeing your child suffering and feeling guilty*'.

Parents found it hard when they felt that their knowledge of their child was ignored: '*The staff at hospital who did not listen to mother*', '*Not having your mothering/fathering instincts listened to*'. Parents suggested that it would be helpful if doctors could talk to them using more accessible language when explaining what is wrong with their child: '*Getting doctors to explain the child's condition in layman terms, not "doctor speak"*'.

Parents also reported significant emotional problems following their child's stroke and suggested that meeting other parents would be very beneficial: *'We have at times both seriously contemplated suicide', 'Parents benefit from meeting other parents'.*

The majority of parents felt that they have to constantly fight public services so their child can receive the care and treatment that they should be getting: *'Having to constantly fight for the justice of your child', 'Having to fight/ask for help when you are so vulnerable'.*

All quotes are from participants in the paediatric stroke workshop.

Communication with the child and their family

The recognition that the child is part of a family is central to paediatric care. Any childhood illness has an impact on the whole family, including parents, siblings and grandparents. Childhood stroke has been shown to have an adverse impact on parents' emotional and physical health (Gordon *et al* 2002).

Stroke is a completely unexpected illness in a child and parents and children feel emotionally devastated by the diagnosis. This is compounded by the lack of awareness of childhood stroke amongst professionals, which means that it is often left to the child and family to pursue treatment, rehabilitation and appropriate educational support. All professionals should be aware of the stress associated with a diagnosis of stroke on the child and family from the outset. The importance of emotional support and sensitive and comprehensive communication at the time of diagnosis of a disorder with potential long-term developmental consequences is emphasised in *Together from the start* (DfES 2002) and the *Standards for child development services* (RCPCH 1999).

The Stroke Association and Different Strokes (see Appendix 4 for contact details) provide information and support for children affected by stroke and their families. Children, family members or carers need both factual and practical information at various stages, presented in a format appropriate to their needs (Rushforth 1999; Helps *et al* 2003). It should be recognised that parents have particular knowledge of their child and, therefore, their concerns should be addressed in planning the child's care and educational placement.

Guidelines

1   Families/carers should be given factual information about their child's condition as soon as possible after diagnosis (**D**). This should be simple and consistent, avoiding technical terms and jargon

2   Written information should be provided to the child and family regarding the child's health and the statutory and voluntary services available (**D**)

3   Children should be given information about their condition at an appropriate level (**D**)

4   The child and family should be involved in making decisions about the child's care, including rehabilitation and education (**D**)

5   The multidisciplinary health team at secondary level should provide co-ordinated care and liaise closely with education and social services through the key worker (**D**)

Evidence

1 Paediatric stroke workshop (**4**); *Together from the start* (DfES 2002) (**4**); *Standards for child development services* (RCPCH 1999) (**4**)

2 *Together from the start* (DfES 2002) (**4**); Paediatric stroke workshop (**4**)

3 Rushforth 2002 (**4**)

4 Report of Bristol enquiry (**www.bristol-inquiry.org.uk**) (**4**); *Together from the start* (DfES 2002) (**4**); *Standards for child development services* (RCPCH 1999) (**4**); *Children's National Service Framework* (DH 2003a) (**www.dh.gov.uk**) (**4**)

5 *Consensus of working party* (**4**); Mukherjee *et al* 1999 (**4**)

5 Acute diagnosis of arterial ischaemic stroke in children

5.1 Definition

The World Health Organization defines stroke as 'a clinical syndrome typified by rapidly developing signs of focal or global disturbance of cerebral functions, lasting more than 24 hours or leading to death, with no apparent causes other than of vascular origin' (World Health Organization 1978). This definition is a *clinical* one and such a presentation has many potential underlying causes in childhood. Brain imaging is mandatory for accurate diagnosis, subsequent referral and, in particular, to exclude conditions requiring urgent neurosurgical intervention. Arterial ischaemic stroke, which is the main focus of these guidelines, can be defined as 'a clinical stroke syndrome due to cerebral infarction in an arterial distribution'. Transient ischaemic attacks (TIAs) (where the neurological deficit resolves within 24 hours) may also occur in children. Although clinical symptoms may be transient, a significant proportion of children with this presentation have cerebral infarction. Terms such as 'acute infantile hemiplegia' are clinical descriptions, which do not identify the underlying aetiology; they should, therefore, be avoided.

The following sections will deal, firstly, with guidelines for establishing a diagnosis in a child presenting with an acute clinical stroke syndrome (section 5.2), and then discuss the further investigation of children with a diagnosis of arterial ischaemic stroke in order to establish underlying aetiology (section 5.3). It may be pragmatic to combine the initial (diagnostic) and subsequent investigations, especially in the case of imaging, and both sections should, therefore, be considered together.

5.2 Presentation and diagnosis

At the time of stroke children and families reported feelings such as 'frightened', 'annoyed', 'angry', 'confused', 'devastated'.

Parents reported feeling concerned and frightened at the amount of time they had to wait for diagnosis, treatment and information about their child's condition: 'Sitting for hours in the emergency department, with ———, before it was finally acknowledged she had had a stroke' (parent participant in paediatric stroke workshop).

Recognition of clinical stroke may be difficult, particularly in infants and young children, and especially as neurological signs may be relatively subtle. If there is doubt, the child should be examined by a senior paediatrician. The most common clinical presentation of clinical stroke in childhood is with acute hemiparesis. Focal signs may be absent in neonates or young infants, in whom seizures may be the only manifestation of clinical stroke. Clinical symptoms and signs of arterial ischaemic stroke may be particularly subtle in children with sickle cell disease, and may be difficult to distinguish from painful crisis or the effects of treatment, for example treatment with opiates. Advice should be sought from a tertiary centre if there is concern about the acquisition and interpretation of imaging studies in a child with clinical stroke.

Guidelines

1   All children with a clinical presentation of stroke should be under the care of a consultant paediatrician ✓

2   Cross-sectional brain imaging is mandatory in children presenting with clinical stroke (C)

3   Brain magnetic resonance imaging (MRI) is recommended for the investigation of children presenting with clinical stroke (C)

4   Brain MRI should be undertaken as soon as possible after presentation. If brain MRI will not be available within 48 hours, computed tomography (CT) is an acceptable initial alternative ✓

5   Brain imaging should be undertaken urgently in children with clinical stroke who have a depressed level of consciousness at presentation or whose clinical status is deteriorating ✓

6   Any new neurological symptoms or signs in children with sickle cell disease should be evaluated as potentially being due to stroke ✓

7   All children with clinical stroke should have regular assessment of conscious level and vital signs ✓

Evidence (Tables 1 and 2)

1   Consensus of working party

2   Ganesan *et al* 2003 (2+)

3   Bryan *et al* 1991 (2+); Kucinski *et al* 2002 (2+); Barber *et al* 1999 (2–); Lansberg *et al* 2000 (2–)

4   Consensus of working party

5   Consensus of working party

6   Consensus of working party

7   Consensus of working party

5.3 Investigations

This section aims to provide some guidance about investigations in the evaluation of a child with arterial ischaemic stroke; it is not, however, intended to be comprehensive. There are many potential risk factors for arterial ischaemic stroke in children and the diagnostic process should be directed towards identifying as many of these as possible. The proportion of patients in whom no risk factors are identified has decreased as understanding of aetiology and investigation methods have improved. There is little information on the diagnostic sensitivity of individual investigations. Although the investigations discussed below should be undertaken in all cases, other investigations may be indicated in individual patients, and should be considered on a case-by-case basis. For a more complete discussion of this topic see Kirkham 1999. A clerking checklist is provided to highlight important aspects of the clinical history and examination.

Transfer to a tertiary centre may be necessary if facilities for definitive imaging or other investigations (eg echocardiography) are not available locally. As mentioned in relation to brain imaging, advice should be sought from a tertiary centre if there is concern about the acquisition and interpretation of paediatric echocardiography.

Non-invasive cerebrovascular imaging with techniques such as MR angiography (Husson *et al* 2003), CT angiography, ultrasound with Doppler techniques or a combination of such modalities can be applied in the first instance, and may be adequate. The existing research on paediatric arterial ischaemic stroke only includes studies limited to visualisation of the arterial vasculature between the distal common carotid artery and the circle of Willis. The value of imaging the aortic arch and its proximal main branches is unknown. It is acknowledged that, in some cases, non-invasive angiographic techniques alone will not provide sufficient information to enable the planning of subsequent management, and in these cases catheter cerebral angiography may also be required. Due to the lack of specific research evidence we have not made more detailed recommendations regarding imaging sequences but a helpful discussion of these can be found in the review article by Hunter (Hunter 2002).

If there are unusual features to the identified infarct, such as the anatomical location, the presence of excessive brain swelling and then the possibility of venous infarction or haemorrhage should be considered. More specific venous imaging investigations may then be applied by the radiologist as necessary. In the first instance, non-invasive options such as MR venography or CT venography are preferred over catheter angiography.

The yield of investigating children with arterial ischaemic stroke for thrombophilia is variable and will depend on factors such as ethnicity. Protein C deficiency and elevated lipoprotein(a) have been shown to be associated with an increased risk of recurrence (Strater *et al* 2002). Although the appropriate preventative treatment in affected patients is unknown, identification of a prothrombotic tendency may have other implications for the child's more general health, for example risk of venous thrombosis. Additional specific investigations to be included when screening for thrombophilia should be discussed with the local haematology service, with consideration of the local prevalence of specific thrombophilia.

The importance of more conventional childhood stroke risk factors in children with sickle cell disease has not been evaluated. The clinical experience of the working party is that these may play a role in some patients and therefore we would not exclude children with sickle cell disease from the recommendations below.

Guidelines

1   Imaging of the cervical and proximal intracranial arterial vasculature should be performed in all children with arterial ischaemic stroke (**C**)

2   Imaging of the cervical vasculature to exclude arterial dissection should be undertaken within 48 hours of presentation with arterial ischaemic stroke ✓

3   Transthoracic cardiac echocardiography should be undertaken within 48 hours after presentation in all children with arterial ischaemic stroke ✓

4   All children with arterial ischaemic stroke should be investigated for an underlying prothrombotic tendency. This should include evaluation for protein C protein S deficiency, activated protein C resistance, increased lipoprotein (a), increased plasma homocysteine, factor V Leiden, prothrombin G20210A and MTHFR TT677 mutations and antiphospholipid antibodies (**C**)

Evidence (Tables 3 and 4)

The papers cited here provide information about risk factors associated with childhood arterial ischaemic stroke, but do not all provide direct information about sensitivity or specificity of specific diagnostic tests in the context of childhood arterial ischaemic stroke.

1   Levy *et al* 1994 (**2+**); Ganesan *et al* 2002 (**2+**); Husson *et al* 2003 (**2+**); Ganesan *et al* 1999 (**3**)

2   Consensus of working party

3   Consensus of working party

4   Nowak Gottl *et al* 1999 (**2+**); deVeber *et al* 1998b (**2+**); Strater *et al* 2002 (**2+**); Subcommittee for Perinatal and Pediatric Thrombosis of the Scientific and Standardization Committee of the International Society of Thrombosis and Haemostasis (**4**)

6 Acute care

This section relates to all aspects of acute care. Medical care, early evaluation of disability and rehabilitation are equally important aspects. These guidelines assume that, as is usual in the United Kingdom, the early care of a child who has had a stroke will be undertaken in a specialist paediatric neurology or general paediatric ward.

The acute medical management of arterial ischaemic stroke can be divided into general care measures and measures aimed at limiting the extent of ischaemic damage or preventing early recurrence. The latter depend on the likely cause of stroke in each case. As with the adult guidelines, treatment of secondary complications or of associated diseases is not considered here.

Early multidisciplinary evaluation is vital to prevent complications and plan rehabilitation. If the child is in an acute paediatric neurology ward, he or she is likely to have access to a multidisciplinary team with expertise in paediatric neurology. However, on a general paediatric ward it may be necessary for any member of the team to seek advice from colleagues in a tertiary centre. There is no specific research relating to the evaluation and management of children affected by stroke, but principles relating to the evaluation and care of children with other acute neurological conditions and, where available, published guidelines have been applied in formulating these recommendations.

6.1 General care measures

There are no studies which have specifically examined the effect of disruptions in homeostasis on stroke outcome in children but we have highlighted the points below based on principles which would be applied to the care of any acutely ill child, as well as from the evidence base in adults affected by stroke.

Guidelines

1 Temperature should be maintained within normal limits (**D**)

2 Oxygen saturation should be maintained within normal limits (**D**)

Evidence

1 Extrapolation from *National clinical guidelines for stroke: second edition* (Intercollegiate Stroke Working Party 2004) (**4**)

2 Consensus of working party; *National clinical guidelines for stroke: second edition* (Intercollegiate Stroke Working Party 2004) (**4**)

6.2 Specific medical treatments

There are no studies specifically examining the efficacy of acute treatments for arterial ischaemic stroke in children. The following recommendations are based on the consensus opinion of the working party.

The use of anticoagulation in children with cardiac embolism is controversial as it involves balancing the risk of precipitating haemorrhagic transformation of the infarct with the potential to prevent further embolic events. The decision may be influenced by the cardiac pathology, time elapsed after the stroke and by neurological and imaging findings. In the absence of any evidence, we were unable to make a general recommendation, but felt that individual patient management should involve senior clinicians in paediatric cardiology and neurology.

The efficacy and optimal dose of aspirin in the treatment of children with acute arterial ischaemic stroke is unknown. The lowest dose recommended for treatment of other paediatric conditions, such as Kawasaki disease, in the paediatric formulary *Medicines for children* (Royal College of Paediatrics and Child Health 2003) is 5 mg/kg/day. This would approximate to the dose (300 mg) recommended for acute treatment of ischaemic stroke in adults (*National clinical guidelines for stroke: second edition*, Intercollegiate Stroke Working Party 2004) and therefore has been recommended below. The lowest effective dose for long-term prophylaxis may be lower, as discussed in the following section. Although children with sickle cell disease have been excluded from the first guideline, aspirin or anticoagulation may need to be considered if other risk factors, for example arterial dissection, are identified in individual patients.

There is currently no evidence to support use of thrombolytic agents such as tissue plasminogen activator (tPA) in the acute treatment of arterial ischaemic stroke in children.

Guidelines

1 Aspirin (5 mg/kg/day) should be given once there is radiological confirmation of arterial ischaemic stroke, except in patients with evidence of intracranial haemorrhage on imaging and those with sickle cell disease ✓

2 In children with sickle cell disease and arterial ischaemic stroke:

   i   urgent exchange transfusion should be undertaken to reduce HbS to <30% and raise haemoglobin to 10–12.5 g/dl ✓

ii if the patient has had a neurological event in the context of severe anaemia (eg splenic sequestration or aplastic crisis), or if exchange transfusion is going to be delayed for more than four hours, urgent top-up blood transfusion should be undertaken ☑

3 Providing there is no haemorrhage on brain imaging, anticoagulation should be considered in children with:

i confirmed extracranial arterial dissection associated with arterial ischaemic stroke ☑

ii cerebral venous sinus thrombosis (**C**)

4 The decision to use anticoagulation in children with arterial ischaemic stroke who have a cardiac source of embolism should be discussed with a consultant paediatric cardiologist and paediatric neurologist ☑

5 Early neurosurgical referral should be considered in children with stroke who have depressed or deteriorating conscious level or other signs of raised intracranial pressure ☑

Evidence (Table 5)

1 Working party consensus

2 Working party consensus

3 i) Working party consensus; ii) Extrapolation from Stam *et al* 2003 (1–) (level of recommendation downgraded from B to C due to small number of studies in Cochrane review (n = 2) and based on adult data)

4 Working party consensus

5 Working party consensus

6.3 Secondary prevention of arterial ischaemic stroke in childhood

Child in paediatric stroke workshop: 'What happens if you get two strokes?'

Stroke recurrence is a major concern for children and their families. Arterial ischaemic stroke recurs in between 6% and 20% of all children and in over 60% of children with sickle cell disease. The risk of recurrence is increased in children with multiple risk factors (Lanthier *et al* 2000) and in those with protein C deficiency, increased levels of lipoprotein (a) and vascular disease (Sträter *et al* 2002). At present, there is very little evidence regarding the efficacy of secondary prevention strategies (Sträter *et al* 2001) but this is likely to change as the need for multicentre trials is gaining momentum. Thus we would emphasise that the consensus statements below are not long-term recommendations and will need to be updated as new evidence emerges.

Although widely used, the dose of aspirin to be used for secondary prevention of ischaemic stroke is undefined in childhood. Doses between 50–300 mg/day are recommended for adults (*National clinical guidelines for stroke: second edition* Intercollegiate Stroke Working Party 2004) and doses between 1–3 mg/kg/day have been recommended for secondary prevention in children (Nowak-Gottl *et al* 2003). Given the lack of evidence we have not been able to recommend a specific dosage; however, complications such as bruising may limit the dose which can be tolerated by the child.

Guidelines

1 Patients with cerebral arteriopathy other than arterial dissection or moyamoya syndrome or those with sickle cell disease should be treated with aspirin (1–3 mg/kg/day) ☑

2 Anticoagulation should be considered:

   i until there is evidence of vessel healing, or for a maximum of six months, in patients with arterial dissection ☑

   ii if there is recurrence of arterial ischaemic stroke despite treatment with aspirin ☑

   iii in children with cardiac sources of embolism, following discussion with the cardiologist managing the patient ☑

   iv until there is evidence of recanalisation or for a maximum of six months after cerebral venous sinus thrombosis ☑

3 In children with sickle cell disease:

   i regular blood transfusion (every three to six weeks) should be undertaken to maintain the HbS% <30% and the Hb between 10–12.5 g/dl (**C**)

   ii transfusion may be stopped after two years in patients who experienced stroke in the context of a precipitating illness (eg aplastic crisis) and whose repeat vascular imaging is normal at this time (**C**)

   iii after three years a less intensive regime maintaining HbS <50% may be sufficient for stroke prevention (**C**)

   iv those who cannot receive regular blood transfusions because of allo-immunisation, auto-antibody formation, lack of vascular access or non-compliance with transfusion or chelation may be considered for treatment with hydroxyurea (**C**)

4 Children with moyamoya syndrome (including those with sickle cell disease) should be referred for evaluation to a centre with expertise in evaluating patients for surgical revascularisation (**D**)

5 Children with sickle cell disease who have had a stroke should be referred to a specialist centre for consideration of bone marrow transplantation (**B**)

6 Advice should be offered regarding preventable risk factors for arterial disease in adult life, particularly smoking, exercise and diet (**D**)

7 Blood pressure should be measured annually to screen for hypertension ✓

8 Patients who are found to have a prothrombotic tendency should be referred to a haematologist ✓

Evidence (Tables 6, 7, 8 and 9)

1 Consensus of working party

2 Consensus of working party

3 i) Powars *et al* 1978 (**2−**); Portnoy & Herion 1972 (**2−**); Balkaran *et al* 1992 (**2−**); Wilimas *et al* 1980 (**2+**); Russell *et al* 1984 (**2+**); Wang *et al* 1991 (**2+**); Cohen *et al* 1992 (**2+**); De Montalambert *et al* 1999 (**2−**); Rana *et al* 1997 (**2−**); Pegelow *et al* 1995 (**2−**); Scothorn *et al* 2002 (**2+**); Dobson *et al* 2002 (**2+**); ii) Dobson *et al* 2002 and Scothorn *et al* 2002 (**both 2+**); iii) Cohen *et al* 1992 (**2+**); iv) Ware 1999 (**2+**); Sumoza 2002 (**2+**)

4 Golby *et al* 1999; Olds *et al* 1987; George *et al* 1993; Ishikawa *et al* 1997; Matsushima *et al* 1992; Fryer *et al* 2003 (**all 3**)

5 Vermylen *et al* 1998; Bernaudin 1999; Walters *et al* 2000 (**all 2++**)

6 Consensus of working party; Extrapolation from *National clinical guidelines for stroke: second edition*, Intercollegiate Stroke Working Party 2004 (**4**)

7 Consensus of working party

8 Consensus of working party

6.4 Early disability assessment and management

The philosophy of paediatric medicine is for care to be delivered, where possible, in the child's home environment and to minimise the time a child spends in hospital. The inpatient period may be limited to the time when the child is acutely unwell or when there are outstanding diagnostic issues. It is, therefore, important that links to community child health services should be made from the outset in order for a package of care to be set up, and that the child is not discharged until this is in place. Ultimately this package may be delivered in a variety of settings, as discussed in chapter 3. Parents (and children when possible and appropriate) should be involved in planning long-term care.

Guidelines

1 As soon as possible after admission, following stroke all children should have an evaluation of:

i   swallowing safety (**D**)

ii feeding and nutrition ✓

iii communication (**D**)

iv pain (**D**)

v moving and handling requirements (**D**)

vi positioning requirements ☑

vii risk of pressure ulcers (**D**)

2 All children affected by stroke should have a multidisciplinary assessment within 72 hours of admission to hospital ☑

3 The professionals involved in the acute assessment and management of the child should initiate early liaison with their counterparts in the community to ensure a smooth transition of care ☑

Evidence (Table 10)

1 i) Swallowing guidelines of the Royal College of Speech and Language Therapists (RCSLT 2004) (**4**); Morgan *et al* 2003 (**3**); ii) Working party consensus; iii) RCSLT guidelines on assessment of acquired childhood aphasia from the RCSLT's *Communicating quality (2)* (RCSLT 2001) (**4**); iv) Royal College of Nursing's *Clinical Practice Guidelines: The recognition and assessment of acute pain in children* (RCN 2001) (**IV**); v) Royal College of Nursing's *The guide to the handling of patients: fourth edition* (RCN 1999) (**4**); vi) Working party consensus; vii) NICE guideline on pressure ulcer risk management and prevention (Guideline B) (**4**); *Working together to prevent pressure ulcers – a guide for patients and their carers* (**www.nice.org.uk/pdf/clinicalguidelinepressuresoreguidance nice.pdf**) (**4**); *Pressure relieving devices – CG7* (**www.nice.org.uk/pdf/clinicalguidelines pressuresorespatleaftenglish.pdf**) (**4**)

2 Working party consensus

3 Working party consensus

7 Approaches to rehabilitation

Parent in paediatric stroke workshop: 'When we came home from hospital it was as if you're home now – "Goodbye and get on with it". That's the way I feel and still feel. There's been no physio or occupational therapy yet and she's been home about eight weeks now. All I've had is phone numbers and names which are no help to me as there's very little for younger people with strokes. They don't cater for younger children only adults. So it feels as if you're forgotten.'

Parent in paediatric stroke workshop: 'After we came out of hospital the real problems began. The local hospital had little experience of strokes in children. We waited six weeks for physio locally, eight weeks for the OT to assess her. The problem seemed to be "resources" – or shall we say "Government funding"!'

Early rehabilitation of children with acquired brain injury is usually undertaken from the time of diagnosis in the setting of the acute ward; however, subsequent rehabilitation is usually carried out in the community or, in some cases, may be undertaken in a specialist children's rehabilitation unit or on a general paediatric ward (see chapter 3). As previously stated, early liaison and communication between the professionals involved in rehabilitation from tertiary through to primary care services is critical to smooth transition. Rehabilitation interventions may include both 'hands-on' intervention and equipment provision, thus involving a variety of health professionals, education and social services agencies.

The impairments experienced by children affected by stroke, and their functional consequences, may evolve over time due to ongoing growth and development. Rehabilitation of children with limitation in functional skills requires consideration of the impact of sensory, perceptual, motor and cognitive impairments on the individual so that interventions are appropriate. The child and family should be encouraged to express their main concerns about re-integration to the home, community and school environments, and to have these concerns addressed. The impact of stroke on the psychological well-being of the family may adversely affect the child's rehabilitation process. The rehabilitation professional should consult with specialist acute and community-based rehabilitation teams if this is indicated.

There is little evidence on the effectiveness of rehabilitation interventions specifically for children affected by stroke. It may appear in the following sections that there is undue emphasis on sensorimotor function; however, this is because there is a wider availability of research in this domain due to work undertaken in children with cerebral palsy. The reasons for including this literature have been discussed in the introduction. We accept that there are limitations in extrapolating from this population to children with acquired brain injury. Some important differences between the two groups include the level of pre-morbid functioning, age at injury and the rate of change in status. We would also emphasise that, as in children with traumatic brain injury, 'invisible' impairments are under-recognised and a source of significant morbidity in children affected by stroke.

Guidelines

1 Children affected by stroke should be offered advice on, and treatment aimed to achieve, play, self-care, leisure and school-related skills that are developmentally relevant and appropriate to their home, community and school environment (D)

2 Equipment which is appropriate in meeting rehabilitation aims should be assessed on an individual basis, provided in a timely manner, and regularly monitored by appropriate professionals (D)

Evidence

1 The National Association of Paediatric Occupational Therapists' *Guidelines for good practice* (NAPOT 2000) (4); Association of Paediatric Chartered Physiotherapists *Paediatric physiotherapy guidance for good practice* (APCP, revised 2002) (4)

2 The Audit Commission's *Fully equipped* (Audit Commission 2000/2002) (4)

7.1 Sensorimotor rehabilitation

7.1.1 Underlying approach to sensorimotor therapy

The aim of sensorimotor intervention is to improve motor control and physical independence, and to promote developmentally appropriate functional skills. These principles are practised in most therapy approaches. However, they vary according to the type of stimuli used, the emphasis on task-specific practice and/or the principles of learning which are followed. There is little evidence to support the superiority of one treatment approach over another.

Guidelines

1 Sensorimotor therapies should be practiced within a neurological framework, and complement other interventions to improve functional skills ✓

2 Rehabilitation activities should be task orientated and relevant to the individual's life (C)

3 Therapy should be integrated into the child's daily home and school activities (D)

Evidence (Table 11)

1 Working party consensus

2 Ketelaar *et al* 1997 (2++); Butler & Darrah 2001 (4); Volman *et al* 2002 (2+)

3 The Association of Paediatric Chartered Physiotherapists' *Paediatric physiotherapy guidance for good practice* (APCP, revised 2002) (4); Chartered Society of Physiotherapy *Standards of physiotherapy practice* (Chartered Society of Physiotherapy 2000) (4)

7.1.2 Delivery of sensorimotor therapy

Issues regarding the frequency and intensity of contact with therapists are frequently raised by parents and older children. Play and daily living activities enable practice of functional skills and are, therefore, of therapeutic benefit. Collaborative working between parents, teachers or any other member of the multidisciplinary team can ensure that children are able to practise such activities in all their environments.

Goal-setting in therapy involves identifying measurable objectives of performance which are beyond the child's current abilities, but which are considered achievable and relevant to the child's life. Goal-setting may be a helpful adjunct to therapy, in addressing issues of concern to the child, family and therapists, and in measuring the outcome of intervention, and can be useful to record functional changes.

Guidelines

1   Children should be given as much opportunity as possible to practise skills (C)

Evidence (Table 11)

1   Ketelaar *et al* 2001 (2++); Chartered Society of Physiotherapy *Standards of physiotherapy practice* (Chartered Society of Physiotherapy 2000) (4); Downgraded to C as Ketelaar *et al* 2001 was in children with cerebral palsy

7.1.3 Use of assessment measures

Assessment should aim to document a particular aspect of function, impairment, activity and participation as objectively as possible. This will enable the dissemination of information between professionals and services and facilitate the setting of measurable rehabilitation goals and measurement of progress. A wide range of assessment tools is available for the evaluation of children with neurological disorders, of which many are potentially useful in the evaluation of children affected by stroke. It is not possible to make recommendations regarding specific assessment tools as the most appropriate one will depend on many factors, such as the age and developmental level of the child and the resources and training of the team.

Guideline

1   The assessment tools selected should be appropriate for the child's age and developmental and functional level ☑

2   Standardised and validated assessment tools should be used where possible ☑

Evidence

1 & 2 Consensus of working party

7.2 Motor impairment

Both central and peripheral components of motor impairment require consideration during rehabilitation. Hemiparesis is the most common pattern of motor impairment resulting from ischaemic stroke. Spasticity is also common; however, as the basal ganglia are commonly affected in childhood stroke, dystonia or a mixed pattern are seen frequently as well. Hemi-dystonia may have a delayed onset and may follow a period of initial good recovery after the stroke. The upper limb, particularly the hand, tends to be more severely affected than the lower limb in children with ischaemic stroke.

There are a wide variety of treatment interventions available to children with motor impairments but not all have a strong evidence base. These include therapies such as lycra splinting, inhibitive casting, treadmill training, constraint-induced movement therapy and functional electrical stimulation. However, this does not suggest that these treatments are not beneficial if used appropriately. The following guidelines are based on the interventions with an evidence base to support their use.

7.2.1 Muscle strengthening

Muscle weakness is now recognised as a component of disability and studies show that strength training does not increase spasticity and may, in fact, reduce it. Programmes to improve children's muscle strength can lead to improved functional skills. Muscle shortening may also be linked with muscle weakness and interventions which immobilise muscles should be evaluated in terms of their impact on muscle strength.

Guidelines

1 Muscle strengthening should be used as part of the therapy programme to prevent or reverse contractures (**D**)

2 Muscle strengthening activities should be used to improve functional activity (**D**)

Evidence (Table 12)

1 Shortland *et al* 2002 (2+); Downgraded as study of children with cerebral palsy

2 Ross & Engsberg 2002 (2+); Damiano & Abel 1998 (2+); Downgraded as study of children with cerebral palsy

7.2.2 Management of spasticity

Botulinum toxin is a drug used in the treatment of spasticity. It is only effective on the dynamic component of muscle shortening and will not improve fixed contractures. Botulinum toxin is generally safe, has minimal side effects and can be targeted at individual muscles. However, it is an expensive intervention and its effects may reverse after three months. The long-term effects of repeated injections in children are not known. Its potential benefits are enhanced and maintained by concurrent therapy interventions. Currently there are no reliable conclusions on the use of botulinum toxin but a number of studies are underway.

Guidelines

1 If spasticity results in functional limitation or discomfort, botulinum toxin injection may be used to reduce muscle tone and improve range of joint motion (**B**)

2 The most effective dose for gastrocnemius injection is 20 u/kg to reduce the dynamic component of muscle shortening and increase active length (**C**)

3 Botulinum toxin should not be used in isolation from other therapy interventions ✓

Evidence (Table 14)

1 Ade-Hall *et al* 2003 (**1+**) found no strong evidence for or against treatment with botulinum toxin in children with cerebral palsy; Working party consensus

2 Baker *et al* 2002 (**2++**); Downgraded as not specific to this population

3 Working party consensus

7.2.3 Ankle-foot orthoses

The use of ankle-foot orthoses (AFOs) may be considered in children with lower limb involvement. AFOs provide intimate control of the foot and ankle. They are used to maintain muscle length and improve gait patterns. Rigid and hinged AFOs extend to just below the knee with the latter being hinged to allow a limited range of ankle movement. Dynamic ankle-foot orthoses (DAFOs) have a contoured foot support and extend to just above the ankle. Continuous use of rigid orthoses may be implicated in reduced strength of the lower leg muscles.

Guideline

1 A rigid AFO could be considered to aid standing balance, swing through in gait and prevention of foot and ankle contractures ✓

2 A hinged or posterior leaf spring AFO should be used to facilitate normal gait patterns (**D**)

Evidence (Table 13)

1 Consensus of working party (**IV**)

2 Romkes & Brunner 2002 (**2+**); Ounpuu *et al* 1996 (**2−**); Brunner *et al* 1998 (**2+**); Desloovere *et al* 1999 (**2−**)

7.3 Sensory impairment

Clinical experience suggests children may experience disturbance of a variety of sensory modalities following stroke. Some of these may be more easily detectable than others, but all should be considered by health professionals assessing and working with the child as they have the potential to impact outcome and response to rehabilitation.

7.3.1 Somatosensory impairment

Clinical experience suggests that there may be transient or long-term alterations in tactile, proprioceptive and kinaesthetic awareness following childhood stroke. These difficulties may influence movement performance and sensorimotor rehabilitation. They may also influence body awareness and have implications for safety in functional daily activities. Somatosensory assessment relies on careful clinical observation in the absence of accepted valid assessment methods.

Guideline

1   Rehabilitation professionals should consider the presence of somatosensory impairment and integrate this in planning and implementing rehabilitation

Evidence

1   Consensus of working party

7.3.2 Hearing and vision impairment

There is no data on the incidence of vision or hearing impairment in children affected by stroke; however, as with any acquired brain injury, these are potential consequences. Assessment should be comprehensive and include evaluation of both perception and processing of visual and auditory stimuli.

Guideline

1   Vision and hearing should be assessed as part of the multidisciplinary assessment ✓

Evidence

1   Consensus of working party

7.3.3 Pain

Some children reported extreme pain at the time of stroke, for example one child at the workshop reported that when they had the stroke they felt pain which was 'Awful, immense, thousand daggers in my eye, horrible, terrifying'.

Potential sources of pain after childhood stroke include headache, shoulder pain, dysaesthesia and abdominal pain due to gastro-oesophageal reflux. Shoulder pain in adults has been particularly associated with a prolonged hospital stay and poor recovery of arm function, and clinical experience with children would support this. Proprioceptive dysfunction may involve the whole body. Staff should be aware that children may experience pain and discomfort due to sensory disturbance, but can have difficulty expressing this.

Guidelines

1   Children affected by stroke should be assessed for the presence of pain using a validated paediatric pain tool (**D**)

2   All pain should be treated actively, using appropriate measures including positioning, handling, and medication ☑

3   In cases of intractable pain, the child should be referred to health professionals with specialist expertise in pain management ☑

Evidence

1   The Royal College of Nursing's *Clinical practice guidelines: the recognition and assessment of acute pain in children* (RCN 2001) (**4**)

2 & 3 Consensus of working party

7.4 Language and communication

The effects of childhood stroke on language and communication may be specific or global and short- or long-term. Stroke may impair function at any stage of language input (receptive aphasias), language processing (word-finding problems, grammatical problems and other aphasias), speech production (dysarthria) and written language (dyslexia). There may also be problems of social interaction and the willingness to communicate (mutism). Unlike in adults, speech, language and communication consequences may not be determined by which hemisphere is affected and is seen in children with both cortical and subcortical injuries. The child's ability to communicate may also be adversely influenced by physical and/or behavioural problems, their general health, other aspects of their environment (for example, volume of ambient noise) or cognitive skills. Developmental speech and language problems may have been present prior to the stroke and these will need to be taken into consideration when planning management.

Communicating quality (2) (RCSLT 2001) states that a child with communication difficulties requires comprehensive assessment, and that where indicated a specialist speech and language therapist should be responsible for this. Whilst dramatic patterns of recovery have been documented in the early stages of rehabilitation, the prospect of long-term residual deficits, sometimes of a subtle or high level nature, should not be overlooked (Lees & Neville 1990, Lees 1997). Because language learning goes on through the first two decades of life, and the child needs to accommodate to the changing demands of different communication situations, difficulties may surface some time after the initial stroke.

Where children have restricted verbal output or are non-verbal following stroke, the use of alternative and augmentative communication (AAC) systems should be considered. This may include signing, symbols and simple or complex speech output devices. A useful reference is the Communication Matters website (**www.communicationmatters.org.uk**).

Guidelines

1 Professionals working with children affected by stroke should be aware that language and communication skills may be affected (**D**)

2 If parents, professionals or the child's educational assessment raise concerns regarding language or communication, the child should be referred to a specialist speech and language therapist (**D**)

3 A detailed assessment of the child's communication abilities should be carried out in collaboration with the child, parents/carers, teachers and other therapists to identify the child's strengths and weaknesses and plan intervention that aims to increase functional abilities (**D**)

4 A collaborative approach to the management of communication difficulties that includes working with an educational psychologist, other therapists, teachers and social workers should aim to equip the child with a language for life (**D**)

Evidence

1 Lees 1997 (**4**)

2, 3 & 4 *Communicating quality (2)* (RCSLT 2001) (**4**)

7.5 Cognitive effects

The cognitive consequences of stroke in childhood are often underestimated, yet they can impact on all aspects of functioning. Cognitive impairment is particularly likely to be underestimated in children without a physical disability and these children may be incorrectly perceived as not being disabled. Childhood stroke is known to affect both global and specific aspects of cognitive function. The severity of cognitive impairment associated with stroke is variable and, additionally, its impact has to be viewed in a developmental context. Unlike adults, cognitive consequences are not only determined by which hemisphere is affected. They may result from both cortical and subcortical injuries, although limited evidence suggests they are greatest in children with large lesions. Deficits have been reported in intellectual functioning, language and verbal abilities, visual-motor and visual-spatial processing, performance, sequential memory and academic achievement. Specific patterns of impairment may be related to the underlying aetiology or site of injury and, additionally, may emerge during development. For example, attention and executive functioning difficulties have been found in children with sickle cell disease and stroke as these children are vulnerable to frontal lobe damage. Although the child's functioning may still be within the normal range after a stroke, there may be a significant reduction in cognitive functioning and the child's ability to access the curriculum may be altered. Computer-assisted learning may need to be considered to help the child access the curriculum, alongside other specialist interventions.

Cognitive impairment will impact on all aspects of daily functioning. Schools and teachers need to be aware of the potential for cognitive difficulties as these may not be apparent unless the child has a comprehensive assessment. Such an assessment should be carried out in collaboration with colleagues in educational and therapy services and should generate explicit recommendations to support the child both at home and at school. Studies of children with traumatic brain injury suggest that such injury affects the ability of the child to acquire new knowledge; this is also likely to apply to children affected by stroke. Developmental factors, as well as the changing expectations of the child, mean that the functional and educational impact of cognitive impairment is likely to change as the child gets older and therefore their cognitive functioning will need to be reviewed over time.

Children with sickle cell disease are at risk of progressive cognitive dysfunction due to the high incidence of stroke recurrence and 'silent' cerebral infarction. Services for these children should consider repeating cognitive assessments; however, there is no evidence on which to base recommendations about the frequency with which they should take place and the problems of repeated assessment should be considered.

Guidelines

1 Professionals working with children affected by stroke should be aware that cognitive function may be affected, both immediately and in the longer term (C)

2 A detailed psychological assessment of the child's cognitive and functional abilities together with any wider family concerns should be carried out in collaboration with the child, parents/carers and teachers to identify any special educational needs (D)

3 Cognitive assessment should take account of the presence of any visual or hearing deficits ✓

Evidence (Table 15)

1 De Schryver *et al* 2000 (2+); Delsing *et al* 2001 (2+); Kral *et al* 2001 (4); *Access to education for children and young people with medical needs* (DfES 2001) (4)

2 Working party consensus; Paediatric stroke workshop (4); *Access to education for children and young people with medical needs* (DfES 2001) (4)

3 Working party consensus

7.6 Mood and behaviour

Parent in paediatric stroke workshop: 'Because the brain is affected the child is in need of help physically, emotionally and mentally. They often are not the same people they were before the stroke. The parents cannot be expected to cope without the help of experts and the child/teenager definitely benefits if their parent is not always around as family tension/fears can be the cause of much distress at the time.'

Parent in paediatric stroke workshop: 'My daughter also heard voices in her head after her stroke telling her the most distressing things. Stuff that made her feel anxious, guilty and afraid. She felt that her whole life had been turned upside down and that she was going mad. She suffered from severe anxiety attacks, exhaustion and her unhappiness led to a nervous breakdown five years after her stroke.'

There is emerging evidence that childhood stroke has effects on many aspects of behaviour, even in children without apparent difficulties in other domains. There is no specific research on the effects of childhood stroke on mood. However, studies of children with hemiplegia (a group which includes some children affected by acute stroke) has shown that these children experience an increased rate of emotional difficulties (Goodman & Yude 2000). Studies in children affected by stroke have shown that a third of parents feel that their child's behaviour has altered following the stroke (Ganesan *et al* 2000). This observation has been confirmed by a high rate of emotional and behavioural difficulties detected using a behaviour screening questionnaire (Wraige *et al* 2003). In children with sickle cell disease, brain injury is associated with difficulties in decoding emotions and interpreting social situations which may not become evident until adolescence. Unidentified cognitive impairment may exacerbate mood or behaviour problems so both these areas should be evaluated together.

Guidelines

1   Families and professionals should be aware that stroke may have effects on mood and behaviour (**D**)

2   The psychological assessment of the child should include evaluation of mood and behaviour, including wider family concerns (**D**). This should be undertaken in conjunction with cognitive assessment

3   Mood and behaviour should be assessed if there is a change in the child's functioning in the home or school environment ✅

4   If mood or behaviour problems are identified and are having an impact on the child's functioning, the child should be referred to professionals with expertise in treating such problems, such as the local child and adolescent mental health team ✅

Evidence (Table 15)

1   De Schryver *et al* 2000 (2+); Ganesan *et al* 2000 (2+)

2   Boni *et al* 2001 (2+); Max *et al* 2002 (2+); Consensus of working party

3 & 4   Consensus of working party

7.7 Activities of daily living

Motor, sensory and cognitive impairments resulting from a stroke may affect the child's ability to engage in age-appropriate self-care, work and leisure activities. These may include activities such as dressing, bathing, toileting and feeding, and the abilities to move around the home or school environment, play and access the school curriculum. Assessment of the child's ability to perform these activities in the home and school environment is important in facilitating the child's return to community living.

Guidelines

1 Therapists working with a child affected by stroke should assess the child's ability to perform daily living activities ☑

2 An occupational therapist should be involved in identifying therapeutic need in self-care, work/school and leisure activities and provision of intervention in this area if indicated ☑

Evidence

1 & 2 Consensus of working party

8 Longer-term and community care

8.1 Return to school

Parent in paediatric stroke workshop: '——— *has been left both physically and mentally damaged! She is unable to keep up with her peers and my once quite bright little girl is now unable to concentrate, take her studies and pass exams.*'

It is likely that a child affected by stroke will be out of school for a significant length of time. Whilst the child is an inpatient they may attend the hospital school; once discharged, the home teaching service may be involved in provision of education if they are unable to attend school. *Access to education for children and young people with medical needs* (DfES 2001) states that 'all pupils should have access to as much education as their medical condition allows and that each child's situation should be assessed and addressed in a co-ordinated manner by the child's school and the agencies mentioned above'.

The timing of the return to school will vary according to the impact of stroke on the individual child. Return to school is a major milestone in the child's recovery; a positive experience is likely to enhance reintegration. Before the child goes back to school, the local educational authority and school staff should be informed about relevant medical, physical, emotional and cognitive issues. The local education authority is responsible for ensuring that an individually tailored reintegration plan, with multi-agency approval, is in place for all pupils before return to school (*Access to education for children and young people with medical needs* DfES 2001). Although it is important that professionals familiar with the child are involved in liaison, parents should also be encouraged to raise their concerns. Communication is central and this should involve a named teacher (usually the special educational needs coordinator (SENCO)) and the child's key worker.

As the child's physical appearance may have altered as a result of the stroke (for example, if the child has a hemiparesis), staff and pupils should be encouraged to address this in a sensitive manner. The reaction of others to changes in physical appearance is something which many children are apprehensive about and the child should be involved in decisions about how they wish information regarding their illness to be presented to teachers and peers. Children often find it very tiring to return to a full school day after illness, and a graded return to school or the provision of rest periods should be considered. Classrooms are often noisy, with many potential distractions; this may exacerbate problems with attention or concentration. Simple measures, such as changing the child's position in the classroom, may be helpful but should only be undertaken after consultation with the child. Formal therapy programmes should be integrated with the child's school programme.

'Special educational needs' are defined as learning difficulties or disabilities which require special educational provision. The *Special educational needs code of practice* (DfES 2002) and *Special educational needs toolkit* (DfES 2001) clearly outline the steps to identify, assess and meet children's special educational needs. If children require additional input in order to access the national curriculum, the first stages of provision are termed 'School Action' and 'School Action Plus'. The aim of School Action and School Action Plus is to develop individual plans for teaching and learning (termed 'individual education plans'), additional to and different from those usually provided in the child's educational setting, that will enable the child to access an appropriate curriculum. School Action Plus is introduced when changes for School Action have not had sufficient impact on the child's progress. If School Action Plus does not provide appropriate or sufficient support to enable the child to access the curriculum, then a referral can be made to the local educational authority for a statutory assessment of the child's special educational needs, which may lead to a 'statement of educational needs'. If the child's difficulties are very significant from the outset a referral for such an assessment can be made to the local educational authority by the school, parent or by any professional at any stage of the treatment.

Guidelines

1 Child health services, usually community child health services, should take responsibility for informing the local education authority of children who may have special educational needs as soon as possible after the stroke (**D**)

2 The child's key worker should liaise with the special educational needs coordinator at the child's school prior to school return (**D**)

3 A collaborative meeting should be undertaken to plan educational provision with appropriate assessment or support (**D**)

4 Health and school staff should agree procedures for communicating information ☑

5 For children presenting with mobility difficulties, the school environment should be assessed prior to return to school, ideally by an occupational therapist ☑

6 It is recommended that all children affected by stroke are placed on a minimum of School Action (see above) as many difficulties remain latent ☑

Evidence

1 *Special educational needs code of practice* (DfES 2002). Department of Education and Skills 558/2001 (**4**)

2 *Special educational needs code of practice* (DfES 2002). Department of Education and Skills 558/2001; *Special educational needs toolkit* (DfES 2001) (**4**)

3 As above (**4**); *Access to education for children and young people with medical needs* (DfES 2001) (**4**)

4 Consensus of working party

5 Consensus of working party

6 Consensus of working party

8.2 Transition between paediatric and adult services

Childhood stroke may result in lifelong physical and cognitive impairments. The process of transition from paediatric to adult services will depend on the current and future needs of the individual, and will usually occur between 16 and 19 years of age. However, the exact timing will depend on the individual's needs and should be discussed with the young person and family. Key aspects of transition are the transfer of responsibility for health care and the provision of education, training or employment after leaving school. A coordinated approach is critical and advance planning is essential to ensure smooth handover of any and all aspects. The period of transition is often a difficult time for young people and families. Vulnerable aspects of functioning, such as emotion or cognition, may be adversely affected by the stress associated with this if there is inadequate planning and support.

Children with active medical needs will require transfer of health care. These needs may relate to surveillance and management of an active condition (such as cardiac disease or sickle cell disease), as well as to the management of chronic disability. There are different models of transition (for example transfer from paediatric to adult sub-specialist or co-ordination of transfer by the general practitioner (Tuffrey & Pearce 2003)). The most appropriate model should take the young person's needs, as well as the available services, into consideration. The medical team involved in overseeing the young person's health care needs should be involved in planning and managing the handover of overall medical care. The *Special educational needs code of practice* (DfES 2001) provides information on the processes and agencies which should be involved in planning transition after school for young people with special educational needs. It is recommended that a multi-agency transition plan is developed to facilitate successful transition to post-school education, training or work.

If formal medical and therapy interventions have ceased and new problems attributable to the stroke or its aftermath become apparent, the young person's general practitioner should refer them to an appropriate adult service. The paediatric services previously involved in the young person's care should provide or share information. Primary health care professionals should be aware of the potentially wide-ranging effects of childhood stroke and, as emphasised elsewhere in this document, that functional difficulties may emerge after a 'silent' interval.

Guidelines

1 Paediatric general and specialty clinics and child development services should have a local policy on transition to adult services, which should be the responsibility of a named person (**D**)

2 A named professional should take responsibility for arranging an introduction to adult health services ✅

3 A flexible approach to the timing of this transfer needs to be considered which takes into account the young person's readiness, current health status and links to other social transitions such as leaving school (**D**)

4 A multi-agency transition plan should be formulated for young people with special educational needs, with input from health, education and social services, and the young person, to plan transition into further education, training or employment (**D**)

5 A named professional should take responsibility for co-ordinating the transition plan and ensuring delivery of services (**D**)

Evidence

1 *Standards for child development services* (RCPCH 1999) (**4**)

2 Consensus of working party

3 Children's National Service Framework (**www.dh.gov.uk**) (**4**)

4 *Standards for child development services* (RCPCH 1999) (**4**); *The special educational needs code of practice* (DfES 2001) (**4**)

5 *Special educational needs code of practice* (DfES 2001) (**4**)

9 Primary prevention

As the mechanisms and risk factors for arterial ischaemic stroke in children are not well understood at present, there is no research on effective primary prevention strategies other than in children with sickle cell disease. Although primary prevention of stroke in children in sickle cell disease is possible with regular prophylactic blood transfusion, this has many risks and disadvantages which should be clearly discussed with the child and family.

Guidelines

1 Children with haemoglobin SS or Sβ° thalassaemia should be screened yearly from the age of three years for internal carotid artery or middle cerebral artery velocity >200 cm/s using appropriately trained personnel and transcranial Doppler ultrasound (**B**)

2 Children with sickle cell disease who have internal carotid artery/middle cerebral artery velocity >200 cm/s should be offered long-term blood transfusion (**B**)

Evidence

1 Adams *et al* 1998 (**2++**)

2 Adams *et al* 1998 (**2++**)

Appendices

Appendix 1
Peer reviewers

Child and adolescent psychiatrist

Professor Robert Goodman   King's College Hospital, London

Child neurologist

Dr Gabrielle de Veber   The Hospital for Sick Children, Toronto, Canada

Clinical psychologists

Dr Peter Fuggle   British Psychological Society, Leicester

Ms Annette Lawson   Birmingham Children's Hospital

Ms Dianne Melvin   Great Ormond Street Hospital for Children, London

Dr Arleta Staza Smith   Queen's Medical Centre, Nottingham

Community paediatricians

Dr Moira Dick   Mary Sheridan Centre for Child Health, London

Dr Tom Hutchison   Bath and NE Somerset Primary Care Trust

Education consultant

Ms Beth Wicks   Nottingham

Neuroradiologists

Professor Paul Griffiths   University of Sheffield

Dr Neil Stoodley   Frenchay Hospital, Bristol

Occupational therapists

Ms Jane Galvin   Royal Children's Hospital, Melbourne

Dr Elizabeth White   College of Occupational Therapists, London

Paediatrician (neurology and neurodisability)

Dr Diane Smyth   St Mary's Hospital, London

Paediatric neurologists

Dr Richard Appleton   Alder Hey Children's Hospital, Liverpool

Dr Tony McShane   John Radcliffe Infirmary, Oxford

Dr Keith Pohl   Guy's Hospital, London

Dr William Whitehouse   Queen's Medical Centre, Nottingham

Paediatric neurology nurse specialist

Ms Shona Mackie	Southampton General Hospital

Patient organisations

Mrs Margaret Goose	Stroke Association, London
Mr Keith Wood	Different Strokes, Milton Keynes

Physiotherapists

Ms Shelley Cox	Southampton General Hospital
Ms Lorna Stybelska	Cumberland Infirmary, Carlisle

Speech and language therapists

Ms Lucy Cuthbertson	Southampton General Hospital
Ms Nicola Jolleff	Wolfson Centre, London
Ms Valerie Moffatt	Chailey Heritage School, East Sussex
Professor Bruce Murdoch	University of Queensland, Brisbane

Appendix 2
Proposed audit criteria

These criteria have been proposed by the working party for clinical audit. They are divided into two sections – one dealing with acute care and another with longer-term issues. We recognise the importance of patient (child and family) and public involvement in the audit process (see **www.chi.nhs.uk/eng/audit/index.shtml**). Due to lack of resources it has not proved possible to include this perspective in the proposed criteria but this will be addressed in future editions.

Acute care

1　During acute management:

▸　was the child referred to a consultant paediatric neurologist?

▸　if not, was the management of the child discussed with a consultant paediatric neurologist?

2　How many hours after the onset of acute symptoms did the child undergo brain imaging (includes all children presenting with clinical stroke)?

3　In children with arterial ischaemic stroke what other imaging studies were carried out and when were these done:

▸　MRI brain

▸　MRA circle of Willis

▸　imaging of cervical vessels (any modality)

▸　cardiac echocardiogram?

4　When was the first documented assessment (state hours after admission) by:

▸　a nurse

▸　a physiotherapist

▸　an occupational therapist

▸　a speech and language therapist

▸　a psychologist?

5   Was a member of the community child health team contacted prior to transfer to the community (state number of days before transfer and which professional was contacted)?

6   During the initial admission, was the family provided with written information regarding:

   ▶ childhood stroke

   ▶ statutory and voluntary agencies?

Longer-term care

7   Is the child under the care of a consultant paediatrician? If so, have they been seen in the last 12 months?

8   Is the child on treatment for secondary prevention of stroke?

9   When was the first documented contact (state weeks after transfer home) by:

   ▶ a key worker

   ▶ a nurse

   ▶ a physiotherapist

   ▶ an occupational therapist

   ▶ a speech and language therapist

   ▶ a psychologist?

10 Was a meeting held between professionals in health and education services and the child's parents prior to the child's return to school?

Appendix 3
An example of the ICF

The components of the International Classification of Functioning, Disability and Health (ICF) might be used to describe the health of a nine-year-old boy affected by a right hemisphere ischaemic stroke in the following way.

Body functions and structures

Impairments include i) clinical findings of left sided hyperreflexia, hypotonia and persistent posturing of the left foot and ankle, ii) imaging findings of right middle cerebral artery territory infarction.

Functional and structural integrity includes the ability to swallow, speak and stand independently and the absence of neurological signs in the right side.

Activities and participation

Activity limitations include difficulties transferring from chair to standing and negotiating obstacles when walking. Short-term memory difficulties found on formal testing leading to difficulties in maintaining attention in school, thus affecting school grades.

Activities able to be performed independently may include self-feeding with the right hand, writing, managing buttons one-handed, and conversing with friends.

Participation restriction may include inability to rejoin the school football team (a major source of social contact with friends at weekends) due to running difficulties. Parents may report difficulty being sent on errands independently due to poor memory.

Participation that remains unaffected may include playing computer games with siblings, reading with parents, and going for walks with friends in the neighbourhood.

Contextual factors

Environmental: The child must climb two flights of stairs to reach his class every morning at school. He has difficulty walking quickly, especially when carrying a school bag. This is compounded by the distance between classes and the number of children crowding the corridor. The football coach is hesitant to allow the child to rejoin the football team in case it places him at risk of injury. The boy's friends welcome him back to school, but he not always able to keep up with playground activities and so is sometimes left to play alone.

Personal: The boy does not want to be singled out so does not agree to leaving class earlier than his peers in order to get to the next class on time. His sense of humour enables him to make friends easily, and thus he widens his social network to include other children for more variety of social contact at school.

Appendix 4
Useful addresses

Acquire

Helps children, young people and adults who have an acquired brain injury and face difficulties in learning as a result.

Manor Farm House,
Wendlebury, Bicester,
Oxfordshire OX25 2PW.
Tel: 01869 324339.
Fax: 01869 234683.
Email: **info@acquire.org.uk**
Website: **www.acquire.org.uk**

Afasic

Represents children and young adults with communication impairments, works for their inclusion in society and supports their parents and carers.

2nd Floor, 50–52 Great Sutton Street, London EC1V 0DJ.
Helpline: 0845 355 5577.
Fax: 020 7251 2834.
Email: **info@afasic.org.uk**
Website: **www.afasic.org.uk**

Chest, Heart & Stroke Scotland

Provides advice and support for people in Scotland affected by chest, heart and stroke conditions.

65 North Castle St, Edinburgh EH2 3LT.
Advice line: 0845 077 6000.
Fax: 0131 220 6313.
Email: **adviceline@chss.org.uk**
Website: **www.chss.org.uk**

Children's Brain Injury Trust

Aims to improve the quality of life for all children who have an acquired brain injury (ABI) and to enable them to achieve their full potential.

Child Brain Injury Trust, The Radcliffe Infirmary, Woodstock Road, Oxford OX2 6HE.
Helpline: 0845 601 4939.
Tel: 01865 552 467.
Email: **helpline@cbituk.org**
Website: **www.cbituk.org**

Children's Hemiplegia and Stroke Association

Offers support and information for families of children who have hemiplegia, hemiparesis and/or stroke. Based in the USA.

CHASA Foundation,
Suite 305, PMB 149,
4101 West Green Oaks,
Arlington TX 76016, USA.
Email: **info437@chasa.org**
Website: **www.chasa.org**

Contact a Family

Provides information for families of children with disabilities and/or rare syndromes.

209–211 City Road, London EC1V 1JN.
Tel: 020 7608 8700.
Fax: 020 7608 8701.
Freephone: 0808 808 3555.
Email: **info@cafamily.org.uk**
Website: **www.cafamily.org.uk**

Department for Education and Skills

Provides advice for parents and teachers of children with special educational needs.

Website: **www.dfes.gov.uk/sen**

Department for Work and Pensions

Provides information on a range of benefits and services for families.

Public Enquiry Office
Tel: 020 7712 2171.
Fax: 020 7712 2386.
Website: **www.dwp.gov.uk/ lifeevent/famchild/index.asp**

Different Strokes

For younger people who have had a stroke, mainly young adults. Includes information on access to leisure activities, counselling services, benefits and rights information, and information packs.

Information Officer, Different Strokes, 9 Canon Harnett Court, Wolverton Mill,
Milton Keynes MK12 5NF.
Helpline: 0845 130 7172.
Fax: 01908 313501.
Email:
info@differentstrokes.co.uk
Website:
www.differentstrokes.co.uk

Disability Alliance

Provides information and advice to disabled people and their families about entitlement to social security benefits and services. Publications include the Disability rights handbook.

Universal House,
88–94 Wentworth St,
London E1 7SA.
Tel: 020 7247 8776.
Fax: 020 7247 8765.
Website:
www.disabilityalliance.org

HemiHelp

Provides information and support for children with hemiplegia and their families.

Unit 1, Wellington Works,
Wellington Road, London
SW19 8EQ.
Helpline: 0845 123 2372.
Fax: 0845 120 3723.
Email:
support@hemihelp.org.uk
Website: **www.hemihelp.org.uk**

Independent Panel for Special Education Advice (IPSEA)

Gives free independent advice on education issues, including appealing to special educational needs tribunals.

6 Carlow Mews, Woodbridge,
Suffolk IP12 1EA.
Tel: 01394 380 518.
England & Wales:
0800 018 4016 (freephone).
Scotland: 0131 665 4396
(freephone).
Website: **www.ipsea.org.uk**

The Stroke Association

Provides information and support for people who have had a stroke and their families. Produces wide range of publications, supports research and health education. Provides a national Stroke Information Service and helpline.

240 City Rd, London EC1V 2PR.
Helpline: 0845 3033 100 (local
rate within UK).
Fax: 020 7490 2686.
Email: **info@stroke.org.uk**
Website: www.stroke.org.uk

Sickle Cell Society

Provides information, counselling and caring for those with sickle cell disorders and their families.

54 Station Road, Harlesden,
London NW10 4UA.
Tel: 020 8961 7795.
Fax: 020 8961 8346.
Email:
sickleinfo.line@btinternet.com.
Website:
www.sicklecellsociety.org

Tables of evidence

Table 1 Acute diagnosis and presentation

Source	Design and subjects	Intervention	Outcome measures	Results	Quality and comment
Ganesan et al, 2003	Observational study of 356 children with stroke and description of risk factors encountered in 212 with radiologically confirmed AIS presenting to tertiary referral centre	Description of risk factors encountered; incidental data on diagnoses in patients with clinical stroke subsequently found not to have AIS	–	Nearly 20% of children with stroke had a diagnosis other than AIS. Another 10% had normal imaging	Uncontrolled study; possible referral/selection bias; opportunistic sample

AIS = Arterial ischaemic stroke

Table 2 CT vs MRI in the neuroimaging diagnosis of acute ischaemic stroke

Source	Design and subjects	Intervention	Outcome measures	Results	Quality and comment
Bryan et al, 1991	Observational study; n = 31	CT and MRI performed within 24 hours and at 7–10 days	–	MR appears to be more sensitive than CT in the imaging of acute stroke	Study design favours MRI over CT. Justification by authors in subsequent commentary
Kucinski et al, 2002	Observational study; n = 25	Quantification of diffusion changes on MRI against density changes on CT in acute stroke	Diffusion (MRI) changes by 21%. Density (CT) changes by 4%	Provides technical evidence to explain the lower sensitivity of CT compared with MRI for detection of early ischaemic changes in imaging studies	Objective support for previous subjective observational studies that show MRI being advantageous over CT (see below)
Barber PA et al, 1999	Observational study; n = 17	Identification of major ischaemia and association with outcome	–	DWI is more sensitive than CT in the identification of acute ischaemia and can visualise major ischaemia more easily than CT	Subjective observational study showing MRI being advantageous over CT
Lansberg MG et al, 2000	Observational study; n = 19	Accuracy of early MRI vs CT and correlation with final infarct volume	–	MRI was more accurate for identifying acute infarction and more sensitive. Lesion volume on acute MRI, but not on acute CT, correlated strongly with final infarct volume	Subjective observational study showing MRI being advantageous over CT

CT = Computerised tomography; DWI = Diffusion weighted imaging; MRA = Magnetic resonance angiography; MRI = Magnetic resonance imaging; Obs = Observational study

Table 3 Investigation

Source	Design and subjects	Intervention	Outcome measures	Results	Quality and comment
Ganesan et al, 2003	Observational study of 356 children with stroke and description of risk factors encountered in 212 with radiologically confirmed AIS presenting to tertiary referral centre	Description of risk factors encountered; incidental data on diagnoses in patients with clinical stroke subsequently found not to have AIS	Radiologically confirmed AIS	1. 79% had cerebral arterial abnormalities 2. Significant association between trauma and previous chickenpox and AIS in previously healthy patients 3. Anaemia (40%), risk of hyperhomocysteinaemia (21%) common 4. Echocardiography abnormal in 7% of patients only	Uncontrolled study, not all patients had all investigations; possible referral/selection bias
Nowak-Gottl et al, 1999	Multicentre case controls study of 148 children with AIS and 296 controls	Comparison of the rates of FVL, PT20210, t-MTHFR mutations and protein C deficiency and increased Lp(a) levels in children with AIS and controls	Prevalence rates	Lp(a) >30mg/dL OR 7.2, FVL OR 6, Protein C deficiency OR 9.5, PT20210 OR 4.7, MTHFR TT OR 2.64, For combined risk factors OR 35.75	Increased prevalence of all mutations and especially of combined defects. Establishes association, not causation. The prevalence is likely to be different in other ethnic groups so the generalisability is questionable
DeVeber et al, 1998b	Tertiary centre Canadian population; includes arterial and venous, neonates and older	Evaluated for protein C, S, AT, Plasminogen deficiencies, FVL, lupus anticoagulant and anticardiolipin antibodies	Incidence of thrombophilia	92 patients (73 arterial); 35 had at least 1 abnormality, 25/73 with arterial ischaemic stroke. 23 had anticardiolipin antibodies, 6 had lupus anticoagulant, 10 had AT deficiency, 10 had protein S deficiency, 7 had plasminogen deficiency, 6 had protein C deficiency, 6 had APC resistance, 0 had FVL. No significant difference between neonates and older children	Limited value as mixed population but suggests high incidence of abnormalities in arterial subgroup

continued

Table 3 Investigation *continued*

Source	Design and subjects	Intervention	Outcome measures	Results	Quality and comment
Strater et al, 2002	Multi-centre study, Germany; 324 white children aged 7 months to 18 years at time of first stroke. All radiologically confirmed. Excluded sickle cell. 123 had another diagnosis	All investigated for thrombophilia (protein C, S and AT deficiencies, fV and fII mutations, APC resistance, antiphospholipid antibodies and high Lp(a). Other investigations variable	Stroke recurrence	301 followed up. 20 had recurrence at median of 5 months; fatal in 3. Independent associations with recurrence: protein C deficiency (OR 10.7), Lp(a) >300 mg/L OR 2.8, vascular stroke OR 3.9	Good study but limited by highly selected patients group – applicable to other populations? Thoroughness of investigations other than for prothrombotic states not clear

AIS = Arterial ischaemic stroke; FVL = factor V Leiden; Lp(a) = lipoprotein (a); t-MTHFR = Thermolabile methylene tetrahydrofolate reductase mutation; OR = odds ratio; PT = prothrombin

Table 4 Angiographic imaging following AIS

Source	Design and subjects	Intervention	Outcome measures	Results	Quality and comment
Ganesan et al, 2003	Observational study; n = 212. Paediatric stroke, with cerebral angiography in 185 cases	–	–	Spectrum of cerebrovascular disease identifiable as risk factors in paediatric stroke	Provides guidance for imaging recommendations
Levy et al, 1994	Observational study; n = 19	Comparing MRA against CA in the investigation of dissection. CA used as gold standard	–	MRA performs less well for vertebral dissection	Early paper. Provides some guidance for imaging recommendations
Ganesan et al, 2002	Observational study; n = 22	Radiological findings of posterior circulation stroke in children	–	Many patterns of angiographic abnormality	Provides some guidance for imaging recommendations
Hasan et al, 2002	Review paper	Studies of vertebral dissection in children	–	Indicates poor results for MRA	Summary of the imaging issues. Provides some guidance for imaging recommendations
Ganesan et al, 1999	Retrospective review of angiographic results in paediatric stroke; n = 46	Angiography	–	Indicates high prevalence of abnormalities and added value of catheter angiography in selected cases	Provides some guidance for imaging recommendations

continued

Table 4 Angiographic imaging following AIS continued

Source	Design and subjects	Intervention	Outcome measures	Results	Quality and comment
Husson et al, 2003	Diagnostic observational; n = 24 children with ischaemic stroke	MRA vs contrast angiography	No. of lesions	MRA found all major lesions. No normal cases missed. MRA is sensitive enough to give initial evaluation of arterial brain disease in children (non-invasively)	Reasonable study, rather limited sample

MRA = Magnetic resonance imaging

Table 5 Acute treatment

Source	Design and subjects	Intervention	Outcome measures	Results	Quality and comment
Stam et al, 2003	Cochrane review. 2 studies with n = 79; one with standard heparin (n = 20) and the other with LMW heparin	Effectiveness and safety of anticoagulation in patients with cerebral venous sinus thrombosis	Death, death or dependency, bleeding and thrombotic complications	Anticoagulation associated with relative risk of death 0.33 (0.08, 1.21) and of death/dependency 0.46 (0.16, 1.31). One GI haemorrhage in treated group and 2 PE in controls	Non-significant reduction in death or dependency; based on small numbers from 2 studies

GI = Gastrointestinal; LMW = Low molecular weight; PE = Pulmonary embolism

Table 6 Revascularisation surgery for moyamoya

Source	Design and subjects	Intervention	Outcome measures	Results	Quality and comment
Golby et al, 1999	Qualitative n = 12 (21 hemispheres); paediatric moyamoya	Direct EC-IC (concurrent EDAS in 6)	TIA/stroke recurrence; Radiol (MRI); cerebral blood flow; (Xenon CT)	All improved/stabilised; no new clinical strokes or ischaemic lesions on MRI; improved blood flow	Heterogeneous treatment; mean follow-up 35 months; advocate direct procedure
Olds et al, 1987	Case control (retrospective); n = 23	Surgery 15 (direct 5, indirect 10); no surgery 8	Clinical (subjective); radiology (weak)	No surgery poor outcome. Surgery stabilised or improved	Weak study but some attempt at control. Reasons for no surgery? Conclusion: surgery better than no surgery, direct better than indirect

continued

Table 6 Revascularisation surgery for moyamoya *continued*

Source	Design and subjects	Intervention	Outcome measures	Results	Quality and comment
George et al, 1993	Qualitative; n = 15	Direct 14; indirect 1	Clinical (subjective)	Further stroke 2; further TIA 5 (decreased severity 3); no further events 7; death 1	Qualitative data, uncontrolled, implication direct surgery: -low morbidity -improves natural history
Ishikawa et al, 1997	Qualitative; paediatric n = 34 (64 hemispheres); (study subgroup 23 patients > 5 years follow-up)	Indirect 16 hemispheres; direct + indirect (combined) 48 hemispheres	Clinical (subjective); i) ischaemic events, ii) ADL	Post-op ischaemic deficits; indirect 56%, combined 10%. Long-term follow-up ADL no significant difference between surg groups	Useful retrospective study; favouring direct surgery. Comparable groups?
Matsushima et al, 1992	Retrospective cohort paediatric	Comparison of direct *vs* indirect (7 *vs* 13 hemispheres)	Collateral vessel formation; clinical symptoms	Collateral formation better and clinical improvement better in direct group	One of very few papers to address the issue of 'best technique'; small numbers
Fryer et al, 2003	Columbia, NY cohort of patients with SCD and moyamoya; n = 6. Follow-up mean 33 months (28–43 months)	Encephaloduroarteriosynangiosis	Recurrent clinical event	1/6 had a further event ipsilateral to the EDAS 2 weeks later	Small numbers, no control group

ADL = Activities of daily living; EC-IC = Extra-intracranial; EDAS = Encephaloarteriodurosynangiosis; MRI = Magnetic resonance imaging; SCD = Sickle cell disease; TIA = Transient ischaemic attack

Table 7 Secondary prevention of stroke in sickle cell disease (blood transfusion)

Source	Design and subjects	Intervention	Outcome measures	Results	Quality and comment
Powars et al, 1978	Cohort + 3 referral. 33 SS, 2 SC. First stroke aged 20 months to 36 years. 25 infarct, 1 haemorrhage	None (natural history study with which all others compared)	Recurrent 'episode' in patients with infarct	10/15 (67%) of patients with infarcts had recurrence in childhood	Part retrospective. Endpoint includes strokes + TIAS + ? seizures; no repeat imaging.
Portnoy & Herion, 1972	Columbia Cohort	None	Recurrence	20%	–

continued

Table 7 Secondary prevention of stroke in sickle cell disease (blood transfusion) *continued*

Source	Design and subjects	Intervention	Outcome measures	Results	Quality and comment
Balkaran et al, 1992	Jamaican cohort; n = 13	None	Recurrence	6 (47%) recurrent event	–
Wilimas et al, 1980	Memphis cohort; n = 12; arteriography normal in 2 and abnormal in 10	Transfusion HbS <20% for 1–2 years, 10 then stopped	Recurrent stroke; improvement in arteriography	7/10 patients who stopped transfusion had recurrent stroke. Arteriography did not improve in any	Small numbers
Russell et al, 1984	Children's Hospital of Philadelphia cohort; 34 SS, ISC, 1st stroke aged 18 months – 18 years. Arteriography abnormal multiple stenosis/occlusion	4 patients not transfused; for remainder, if arteriography abnormal transfusion at 3–4 week intervals (Hb >8–10 g/dl, HbS <30%)	Recurrent 'episode'; stroke; RIND; TIA	3/4 patients with multiple arteries affected and not transfused recurred. Transfusion to HbS <30% reduced recurrence from 90% to 10% in patients with multiple arteries abnormal	Well-characterised patients. Intervention clear. Endpoint mixed; no repeat imaging; not generalisable beyond patients with multiple vessel abnormalities
Wang et al, 1991	Memphis cohort n = 10; all cerebrovascular disease. 5 unilateral	Transfusion HbS <30% for 5–12 years (median 9.5 years); then stop	Recurrent events	5/10 recurrent stroke (3 mild ischaemia same territory, 2 massive haemorrhage (1 C/L); 1/10 died; 3/10 declined further tx	Small numbers. All CVD. Developing moyamoya?
Cohen et al, 1992	Philadelphia cohort transfused to HbS <30% for stroke for at least 4 years n = 15	Transfusion to HbS 50%	Recurrent events	2 haemorrhages but at HbS c.30%. No recurrent infarcts	No vascular imaging
De Montalambert et al, 1999	French cohort; n = 19	Transfusion in 9; no transfusion in 10	Recurrent stroke	No recurrence in 10 untransfused	Selection bias?
Rana et al, 1997	Howard cohort, Washington; n = 9 (infarct on CT in 8)	Tx every 3–6 weeks to HbS <30% for median 6 years (range 1.5-16 years), then stopped except in emergency	Recurrent events	Hydroxyurea started in 6 patients for other indications, median 4 years (3/12 to 17 years) later	Patients Rx HU & tx for chest crisis, pain, anaemia, surgery 3.9/y (0–7)

continued

Table 7 Secondary prevention of stroke in sickle cell disease (blood transfusion) *continued*

Source	Design and subjects	Intervention	Outcome measures	Results	Quality and comment
Pegelow et al, 1995	Multicentre cohort. Transfused patients 57 SS, 2 Sβ⁺, 1 Sβ⁰. 1st stroke age 20 months to 24 years	All transfused to HbS <30%	Recurrent stroke with new infarct/haem. Recurrent TIA	Recurrent stroke 4.2/100 patient years; 8 recurrent strokes (2 haemorrhage, both HbS <30%, 6 infarcts, 5/6 HbS >30%). Recurrent TIA in 13: 6 HbS >30%	Clinical definition adhered to. Comparison with historical cohorts. Vascular imaging not mandatory
Scothorn et al, 2002	Multicentre cohort. 1st stroke 1.4–14 years. All SS n = 137. Stroke defined clinically and with imaging	All transfused for at least 5 years at least 6 weekly	Recurrent stroke: acute neurological syndrome – symptoms and signs > 24 hours	31/137 (23%) had at least 1 recurrent stroke. Mean time to recurrence = 4 years. Recurrence 2.2/100 patient years. After 2 years recurrence continued only in those with no antecedent event	Clinical definition. Vascular imaging not reported. Retrospective HbS at time of stroke not available for all but at varying times after 1st stroke
Dobson et al, 2002	Single centre cohort. SS with stroke <18 years 1980–99	Transfusion to HbS <30% for 2.2–20.4 years	Recurrent cerebrovascular event stroke >24h ± imaging. TIA <24h; no imaging	41% had recurrent strokes or TIA. Recurrence commoner in Moyamoya	Clinical definition. Vascular imaging

ICA = Internal carotid artery; MCA = Middle cerebral artery; RCT = Randomised controlled trial; RIND = Reversible ischaemic neurological deficit; SC = Haemoglobin sickle cell disease; SS = Homozygous sickle cell disease; TCD = Transcranial Doppler ultrasound; TIA = Transient ischaemic attack; Tx = Transfusion

Table 8 Secondary prevention of stroke in sickle cell disease (hydroxyurea)

Source	Design and subjects	Intervention	Outcome measures	Results	Quality and comment
Ware et al, 1999	Duke cohort of patients who had been transfused for stroke for at least 2 years but were alloimmunised (n = 2), had autoantibodies (n = 4), had stroke on tx (n = 1), had ferritin> (n = 11) or were non-compliant (n = 5) with blood tx and/or chelation	Hydroxyurea 15 mg/kg/d escalated as tolerated up to max 30 mg/kg/day for 3–52 (median 22 months)	Recurrent stroke	3/16 (19%) patients restroked on hydroxyurea, mainly early before max HbF increase. 1 patient who was non-compliant with hydroxyurea as well as blood had stroke 4 months after stopping	Cohort. Relatively short-term follow-up. No vascular imaging. Some patients did not have vasculopathy so had low risk of restroke?
Sumoza et al, 2002	Valencia, Venezuela cohort n = 5; 1 TIA, 4 stroke. Rx hydroxyurea; 2 after 2nd strokes; 3 - 1st stroke (no Tx)	Hydroxyurea 40 mg/kg/day in 4, 30 mg/kg/day in 1	Recurrent stroke or TIA	None had recurrent event over 42–112 months	Cohort; small numbers; no vascular imaging; parietal infarcts or white matter abnormality. Venous infarcts

Table 9 Secondary prevention of stroke in sickle cell disease (bone marrow transplantation)

Source	Design and subjects	Intervention	Outcome measures	Results	Quality and comment
Vermylen 1998	Belgian BM Tx	HLA-identical stem cell Tx (bone marrow, 48; cord blood, 2)	Survival, disease-free survival	93% survival, 82% disease free	–
Bernaudin 1999	French BM Tx	Bone marrow transplant from HLA-identical siblings	Survival, absence of SCD, recurrent stroke	91% survival, 85% disease free, 1/16 (6%) recurrent stroke	–
Walters et al, 2000	USA BM Tx cohort n = 50 (48 SS); follow up 57.9 months (38–95)	Stem cell transplant c Px phenytoin, control of hypertension, Mg2+ supps if low, Hb 9-11, plt>50,000	Clinical stroke, progression of silent infarction on MRI	94% survival; 84% disease free; no new clinical strokes; MRI stable or improved in all	Short FU; 1 died cerebral haem and 2 GVHD; 9/43 (20%) had seizures soon after BM Tx

BM Tx = Bone marrow transplantation; GVHD = Graft vs host disease; Px = Prophylactic; QALY = Quality adjusted life years; FU = Follow-up

Table 10 Early disability assessment

Source	Design and subjects	Intervention	Outcome measures	Results	Quality and comment
Morgan et al, 2003	Children with TBI presenting to 2 major hospitals in Brisbane; n = 1145 children aged 0–16 years	Incidence characteristics and predictive factors for dysphagia after paediatric traumatic brain injury	Dysphagia	61 patients (5.3%) had dysphagia, 68% severe TBI, 15% moderate TBI and 1% mild TBI ie more severe injury associated with higer incidence of dysphagia. Need for and duration of SALT treatment greater in dysphagic group. Patients with dysphagia likely to have lower GCS and longer need for ventilation	Good study, population based but retrospective

GCS = Glasgow coma score; SALT = Speech and language therapy; TBI = Traumatic brain injury

Table 11 Therapy interventions

Source	Design and subjects	Intervention	Outcome measures	Results	Quality and comment
van der Weel et al, 1991	Matched controls; 7–11 years; 9 hemiplegia; 12 normal	3 conditions of forearm pronation/supination – passive, active no task and active with task	Computerised measures of range of movement	In affected arm 20% increase in range on active movement with task	Good. Implications for assessment and therapy
Law et al, 1991	RCT, 2x2 factorial design. 72 children aged 18 months–8 years with spastic cerebral palsy (quadriplegic or hemiplegic)	Upper limb (UL) inhibitive casting ± intensive or regular neurodevelopmental therapy (NDT), or just regular NDT for 6 month period	Peabody Scales (hand function); QUEST (quality of UL movement); Goniometer (range of movement)	No significant difference between groups in hand function. Casting significant improvement in wrist extension range. Also quality of UL movement improved with casting but decreased post-treatment. Parent compliance important predictor variable	Well designed. Potential confounding factors and influence of external factors considered in analysis. Wide variation however between subjects
Law et al, 1997	RCT randomized crossover. 50 children with cerebral palsy (classification quad, diplegia, hemi), age 18 months–4 years, varying hand function from moderate to severe impairment	4 month intervention (see below), 2 month washout, 4 months other intervention. Intervention either regular OT = 1x week to 1x month or intensive NDT = 1x week + home programme + UL cast = 4 hours/day. Assessment at baseline, 4 months, 6 months and 10 months	Peabody Fine Motor Scales; QUEST; Canadian Occupational Performance Measure (COPM) for parental perception of child's ability in hand activities	No difference hand function, quality of UL movement or parents' perception of child's hand function in either group	Well designed. Effect of therapy vs no therapy input not addressed. As stated by authors, any improvement in function could be due either to developmental progress and/or therapy
Hur 1995	Review of research studies on therapeutic interventions	Various types of therapy interventions NDT, Vojta, vestibular stimulation	Variety	Poorly controlled, small sample sized studies therefore no evidence	No evidence of superiority of any treatment approach
Wright & Granat 2000	Cohort study; 8 children with cerebral palsy, recruited from hospital. Baseline assessment (3 weeks), treatment with FES (6 weeks) and follow-up (6 weeks)	Functional electrical stimulation (FES) for daily 30 minute session	3 sub-tests of Jebsen Hand Assessment; range of wrist movement; strength ('moment') using computer-based tool	Improvement in components of hand function assessed and active wrist extension during treatment block and in follow-up period. No change in wrist extension 'moment' (strength) during treatment block	No control group. Small numbers. Results suggestive of association. Would benefit from larger sample size. Only some components of hand function assessed

continued

Table 11 Therapy interventions *continued*

Source	Design and subjects	Intervention	Outcome measures	Results	Quality and comment
Boyd R et al, 2001	Systematic review; management of upper limb dysfunction in cerebral palsy	Therapies, splinting, casing, medical and surgical interventions	Categorised according to ICIDH-2 (WHO)	Paucity of RCTs. Best evidence for occupational therapy and casting, but small treatment effects	Good summary of literature
Ketelaar et al, 2001	RCT; n = 55 children 2–7 years with cerebral palsy	Functional *vs* NDT	PEDI; GMFM	PEDI showed improvement in functional therapy group. No difference in GMFM	Good
Bower et al, 2001	RCT: 56 children in 2x2 design. Age 3–12. GMCS III & below	Intensive treatment *vs* goal setting	GMFM; GMPM	No significant differences between groups	Good
Butler & Darrah 2001	Review paper	NDT *vs* other types of intervention	Varied	No significant differences found between types of treatment	Good
Volman et al, 2002	12 children with hemiplegia 8–14 years	Comparison of reaching movements with affected and non-affected arm in 3 conditions	Kinematics of movement and movement time	The functional condition demonstrated increased velocity and improvements in smoothness and control	Good
Willis et al, 2002	25 subjects, final number 17; 1–8 years	Cross-over trial; constraint-induced therapy with plaster cast for 1 month	PDMS	Significant improvements between control and treatment conditions	Good, although validity of PDMS not clearly established
Pierce et al, 2002	Single case study; 1 child	Constraint-induced therapy; cotton sling 6 hours per day for 14 days	Jebson Taylor test of hand function, Finger tip force and vertical grip (custom made)	Improved performance times on JTTHF; no consistent changes in precision of movement	Small sample with appropriate measurements

COPM = Canadian Occupational Performance Measure; FES = Functional electrical stimulation; GMCS = Gross Motor Function Classification System; GMFM = Gross Motor Function Measure; GMPM = Gross Motor Performance Measure; JTTHF = Jebson Taylor Test of Hand Function; NDT = Neuro-developmental therapy; PDMS = Peabody Developmental Motor Scales; PEDI = Paediatric Evaluation of Disability Inventory; RCT = Randomised controlled trial

Table 12 Strength training

Source	Design and subjects	Intervention	Outcome measures	Results	Quality and comment
Damiano & Abel, 1998	23 + 9 CP	Measurement of strength and function	Dynamometer; GMFM	Muscle stiffness related to weakness; improved muscle strength correlated with improved GMFM scores	Good
Ross & Engsberg 2002	Retrospective analysis of data	Strength and spasticity test at knee and ankle; 60 children with diplegia, mean age 12 years	Dynamometer	No relationship between spasticity and strength	Good
Shortland et al, 2002	5 adults & 5 children with CP	Ultrasound imaging of gastrocnemius muscle	Decreased muscle fibre diameter in children with CP	Shortening related to decreased muscle fibre diameter and effect on aponeurosis indicating muscle weakness	Good quality: small study on one muscle

CP = Cerebral palsy; GMFM = Gross Motor Function Measure

Table 13 Orthotics

Source	Design and subjects	Intervention	Outcome measures	Results	Quality and comment
Romkes & Brunner 2002	CCT; 12 subjects & 10 controls; hemiplegia	Hinged AFO; DAFO	Gait analysis	Hinged AFO produced a gait cycle closer to normal. Improve heel toe gait and increased stride length compared to DAFO	Good, small sample
Ounpuu et al, 1996	31 children (19 with hemiplegia); crossover design, 2 conditions compared	Use of posterior leaf spring AFO compared to barefoot walking	Gait analysis measuring ankle and foot movement & position	Increased dorsiflexion in terminal and swing phases. No increase in walking velocity	Good
Brunner et al, 1998	14 children; crossover design 3 conditions	Spring type; AFO vs rigid; AFO vs barefoot	Gait analysis	Spring type achieved almost normal rocking of foot, decreased equinus and hip adduction. Rigid AFO re-established heel toe gait. Both better than barefoot	Good
Desloovere et al, 1999	–	Posterior leaf spring vs hinged AFOs	Gait analysis	Increased stride length, improved knee flexion decreased hyperextension	Moderate

AFO = Ankle–foot orthosis; DAFO = Dynamic ankle foot orthosis

Table 14 Botulinum toxin

Source	Design and subjects	Intervention	Outcome measures	Results	Quality and comment
Ade-Hall & Moore 2002	Cochrane Review of BtxA in treatment of lower limb spasticity No. of trials = 3	Botulinum toxin A	Gait analysis; GMFM; 3D gait analysis	No strong evidence for or against	Good; small numbers with short follow-ups; need to address long-term effects and dosage levels
Friedman et al, 2000	32 children, 17 quadriplegia and 14 hemiplegia; 1–18 years	Botulinum toxin A to range of upper limb muscles	ROM and MAS	Improved elbow extension at 1 and 3 months not at 6 months; wrist extension improved at 1 month only; caregiver reported improvement	Poor. Mixed sample; large age range; weak outcome measures
Reddihough et al, 2002	RCT cross-over; n = 49. Mixture of types of CP mainly those at more severe end	Botulinum toxin and physio vs physio alone	GMFM, MAS, joint range and Vulpe Assessment Battery at 3 and 6 months	Minimal changes with significance in 1 or 2 components, limited benefit to functional outcome at 3 and 6 months. Trend to improved fine motor skills on BtxA	Good quality study not specific to stroke or hemiplegia
Baker et al, 2002	RCT double blind	Botulinum toxin at doses of 10, 20, 30 u/kg and placebo to gastrocnemius	Goniometry, active and passive ROM, GMFM at 4, 8 and 16 weeks	20 u/kg most effective dose. Dynamic component of shortening improved at 16 weeks	Good quality. 20 u/kg most effective dose in gastrocnemius. Longer-term study needed

BtxA = Botulinum toxin A; GMFM = Gross Motor Function Measure; MAS = Modified Ashworth Scale; RCT = Randomised controlled trial; ROM = Range of motion

Table 15 Psychology

Source	Design and subjects	Intervention	Outcome measures	Results	Quality and comment
Ganesan et al, 2000	128 with ischaemic stroke; 105 included, 23 not available (moved away, died)	Parental questionnaire; 90 children 3 months–15 years at time of stroke (median 5 years); 22 neuropsychological assessment; MRI scans	Whether impairments interfered with daily life	13 (14%) no residual impairments; 37 (40%) outcome good; 53 (60%) outcome poor. Younger age at time of stroke only significant predictor of adverse outcome. 42% speech and language difficulty; 59% help in school, SEN	Good
Hogan et al, 2000	Review	Intelligence after stroke including hemispheric side of injury, age at injury, locus and extent of lesion, gender and longitudinal effects	–	IQ scores toward lower end of average range but significantly below poplation mean. Lateralisation of intellectual function not evident before 5 years begins to emerge after this and appears to be restricted to preservation of verbal IQ after RH injury. Emphasise need for repeated IQ assessments to determine long-term outcome	Good
De Schryver et al, 2000	Long-term follow-up cohort study 37 children < 16 years. 16 girls, 21 boys	Follow-up 7 years after stroke. Physical check-up, global cognition, QOL measures of physical functional, social and psychological domains	Structured interview; Ravens Progressive Matrices (RPM); WISC-R vocabulary; Card Sorting Test; Denver Devel Screening Test; quality of life questionnaire	RPM slight but statistically signif shift towards weaker performance comp with normal pop. Sig decline in RPM attributed to sub-group with epilepsy. Vocabulary-no shift overall Stat signif relationship between lesion in region of left mid-cerebral artery and low vocabulary. No sig relationship between side and type of lesion. Social functioning negatively influenced by changes in behaviour at home school and with friends. >1/3rd special education; >1/3rd no impairment at mean follow-up of 7 years	–

continued

Table 15 Psychology *continued*

Source	Design and subjects	Intervention	Outcome measures	Results	Quality and comment
Ballantyne et al, 1994	Cohort study; 17 subjects, 8 LH damage (mean age 9 years, 4.1–16.5), 9 RH damage (mean age 11.2 yrs, 4.11–20.10). 17 controls matched for age, sex and SES	–	IQ scores, including VIQ, PIQ	LH group: VIQ, PIQ compromised uniformly. RH group: PIQ most affected, VIQ less affected. LH, RH PIQ equally effected. Compared with controls IQ lower than expected	–
Delsing et al, 2001	Consecutive series, cohort study. 31 children with IAS, 19 male, 12 female. Age of onset 2 months–14.3 years (mean age 4.3 years). 6 children older than 5.11. Time of follow-up 1.6–5.9 years (m = 3.5)	Medical/developmental history and screening. Neurological examination. Parent questionnaire	–	4 children died, 27 (87%) children survived. Of these: 9 (29%) no residual impairment, 9 (29%) mild motor and cognitive impairment, 9 (29%) severe residual impairment, 1/3rd of children attended a school for special education or attended a centre for severe mental disability, 58% recovered or showed mild residual impairment. Large cortical as opposed to sub-cortical location of infarction is a significant risk factor for poor outcome. Young age was not significantly related to poor outcome	–
Kral et al, 2001	General review of neuropsychological aspects of paediatric SCD	Review of the literature on neuropsychological findings from Psych-lit and Medline database (1960–2001). Literature reviewed according to presentation of symptoms with data pertaining to overt CVA, and investigations of more subtle impairment (silent infarcts)	Intellectual functioning, language and verbal abilities, visual-motor and visual-spatial processing, memory and academic achievement	Lesions on right – visual spatial deficits and constructional apraxia. Lesions on the left – relatively greater decrement in language. Deficits in attention and executive function are associated with anterior focal lesions. Growing evidence of impairment in sustained attention and concentration, executive function and visual-motor speed and coordination	–

continued

Table 15 Psychology *continued*

Source	Design and subjects	Intervention	Outcome measures	Results	Quality and comment
Boni et al, 2001	52 children Age 6–17 years with EVA sickle cell disease	Evaluation of learning and behaviour problems; non-verbal emotional decoding abilities; ratings of social emotional functioning	Abbreviated WISC; Diagnostic Analysis of Nonverbal Accuracy (DANVA); Social Skills Rating System; Children's Depression Inventory (CDI); MRI scans	Children who scored lower FSIQ had higher measures on the DANVA subtests. When IQ scores were controlled statistically, results suggest that children with SCD who suffer from documented CNS pathology may encounter difficulty decoding or interpreting certain social situations that are particularly complex or ambiguous	–
Max et al, 2002	Children aged 5–19; 29 stroke; 29 congenital clubfoot, or scoliosis (as controls)	Psychiatric status, cognitive, academic, adaptive and family functioning. Family psychiatric history. Neuroimaging and neurological status	Current psychiatric disorder not present before stroke or orthopaedic disorder (controls)	No significant difference between groups on family function and family psychiatric history. 17/29 (59%) of children with stroke had post condition PD, 4/29 (14%) of orthopaedic controls. 12 (41%) of stroke subjects had a resolved post-medical condition PD 8 (28%) of orthopaedic subjects had resolved post-medical condition PD. Attention deficit/hyperactivity disorder most common (46% post stroke, 17% post orthopaedic). Anxiety disorders – 31% post stroke, 7% post orthopaedic. Mood disorders 21% post stroke, 7% post orthopaedic. Psychiatric co-morbidity common in stroke subjects. Post-stroke PD children higher neurological severity, and seizure activity	–

CNS = Central nervous system; CVA = Cerebrovascular accident; IQ = Intelligence quotient; LH = Left hemisphere; MRI = Magnetic resonance imaging; PD = Psychiatric disorder; RH = Right hemisphere; SCD = Sickle cell disease

References

Adams RJ, McKie VC, Hsu L, Files B *et al* (1998) Prevention of a first stroke by transfusions in children with sickle cell anemia and abnormal results on transcranial Doppler ultrasonography. *New England Journal of Medicine* **339**: 5–11.

Ade-Hall R, Moore A (2003) Botulinum toxin type A in the treatment of lower limb spasticity in cerebral palsy (Cochrane Review). In: *The Cochrane Library,* Issue 3, 2003. Chichester, UK: John Wiley and Sons.

AGREE Collaboration (2001) *The AGREE Instrument.* London: AGREE. The AGREE Instrument is available at: **www.agreecollaboration.org/instrument**

Askalan R, Laughlin S, Mayank S, Chan A *et al* (2001) Chickenpox and stroke in childhood: a study of frequency and causation. *Stroke* **32**: 1257–1262.

Association of Paediatric Chartered Physiotherapists (2002) *Paediatric physiotherapy guidance for good practice.* London: Chartered Society of physiotherapy.

Audit Commission (2000, update 2002) *Fully equipped.* London: Audit Commission.

Baker R, Jasinski M, Maciag-Tymecka I, Michalowska-Mrozek J *et al* (2002) Botulinum toxin treatment of spasticity in diplegic cerebral palsy: a randomized, double-blind, placebo-controlled, dose-ranging study. *Developmental Medicine and Child Neurology* **44**: 666–675.

Balkaran B, Char G, Morris JS, Thomas PW *et al* (1992) Stroke in a cohort of patients with homozygous sickle cell disease. *Journal of Pediatrics* **120**(3): 360–6.

Ballantyne AO, Scarvie KM, Trauner DA (1994) Verbal and performance IQ patterns in children after perinatal stroke. *Developmental Neuropsychology* **10**: 39–50.

Banich MT, Levine SC, Kim H, Huttenlocher P (1990) The effects of developmental factors on IQ in hemiplegic children. *Neuropsychologia* **28**(1): 35–47.

Barber P, Darby D, Desmond P, Gerraty R *et al* (1999) Identification of major ischemic change. Diffusion-weighted imaging versus computed tomography. *Stroke* **30**: 2059–2065.

Bernaudin F (1999) [Results and current indications of bone marrow allograft in sickle cell disease]. *Pathologie et Biologie* **47**(1): 59–64.

Boni LC, Brown RT, Davis PC, Hsu L, Hopkins K (2001) Social information processing and magnetic resonance imaging in children with sickle cell disease. *Journal of Pediatric Psychology* **26**: 303–319.

Bower E, Michell D, Burnett M, Campbell M, McLellan D (2001) Randomized controlled trial of physiotherapy in 56 children with cerebral palsy followed for 18 months. *Developmental Medicine and Child Neurology* **43**: 4–15.

Boyd RN, Pliatsios V, Starr R, Wolfe R, Kerr GH (2000) Biomechanical transformation of the gastroc-soleus muscle with botulinum toxin A in children with cerebral palsy. *Developmental Medicine and Child Neurology* **42**: 32–41.

Boyd R, Morris M, Graham H (2001) Management of upper limb dysfunction in children with cerebral palsy: a systematic review. *European Journal of Neurology* **8** (**Suppl 5**): 150–166.

Bristol Royal Infirmary Inquiry (2003) Learning from Bristol: the report of the inquiry into children's heart surgery at the Bristol Royal Infirmary 1984–1995. London: Department of Health.

Brunner R, Meier G, Ruepp T (1998) Comparison of a stiff and a spring-type ankle-foot orthosis to improve gait in spastic hemiplegic children. *Journal of Pediatric Orthopedics* 18: 719–26.

Bryan R, Levy L, Whitlow W, Killian J *et al* (1991) Diagnosis of acute cerebral infarction: comparison of CT and MR imaging. *American Journal of Neuroradiology* 12: 611–620.

Butler C, Darrah J (2001) Effects of neurodevelopmental treatment (NDT) for cerebral palsy: an AACPDM evidence report. *Developmental Medicine and Child Neurology* 43: 778–790.

Charles J, Lavinder G, Gordon AM (2001) Effects of constraint-induced therapy on hand function in children with hemiplegic cerebral palsy. *Pediatric Physical Therapy* 13: 68–76.

Chartered Society of Physiotherapy (2000) Standards of physiotherapy practice. London: Chartered Society of Physiotherapy.

Cohen AR, Martin MB, Silber JH, Kim HC *et al* (1992) A modified transfusion program for prevention of stroke in sickle cell disease. *Blood* 79(7): 1657–1661.

Damiano DL, Abel MF (1998) Functional outcomes of strength training in spastic cerebral palsy. *Archives of Physical Medicine and Rehabilitation* 79: 119–125.

De Montalembert M, Begue P, Bernaudin F, Thuret I *et al* (1999) Preliminary report of a toxicity study of hydroxyurea in sickle cell disease. French Study Group on Sickle Cell Disease. *Archives of Disease in Childhood* 81(5): 437–9

De Schryver EL, Kappelle LJ, Jennekens-Schinkel A, Boudewyn P (2000) Prognosis of ischemic stroke in childhood: a long-term follow-up study. *Developmental Medicine and Child Neurology* 42: 313–318.

Delsing B, Catsman-Berrevoets C, Appel I (2001) Early prognostic indicators of outcome in ischemic childhood stroke. *Pediatric Neurology* 24: 283–289.

Department of Education (2001) *Special educational needs code of practice and toolkit.* London: Department of Education and Skills.

Department for Education and Skills (2001) *Access to education for children and young people with medical needs.* London: Department for Education and Skills.

Department for Education and Skills (2002) *Together from the start.* London: Department for Education and Skills.

Department of Health (2003a) *Children's national service framework.* London: Department of Health.

Department of Health (2003b) *Every child matters.* London: DH.

DeVeber *et al* (1998a) Anticoagulation therapy in pediatric patients with sinovenous thrombosis. *Archives of Neurology* 55: 1533–1537

DeVeber *et al* (1998b) Prothrombotic disorders in infants and children with cerebral thrombo-embolism. *Archives of Neurology* 55: 1539–1543.

Desloovere K, Huenaerts C, Molenaers G, Eyssen M, De Cock P (1999) Effects of ankle foot orthoses on the gait of cerebral palsy children. *Gait and Posture* 10: 90

Dobson S, Holden K, Nietert P, Cure J, Laver J (2002) Moyamoya syndrome in childhood sickle cell disease: a predictive factor for recurrent cerebrovascular events. *Blood* 99: 3144–3150.

Friedman A, Diamond M, Johnston MV, Daffner C (2000) Effects of botulinum toxin A on upper limb spasticity in children with cerebral palsy. *American Journal of Physical Medicine Rehabilitation* 79: 53–9, 75–8, 99.

Fryer RH, Anderson RC, Chiroboga CA, Feldstein NA (2003) Sickle cell anemia with moyamoya disease: outcomes after EDAS procedure. *Pediatric Neurology* 29: 124–130.

Fullerton H, Chetkovich D, Wu Y, Smith W, Johnston S (2002) Deaths from stroke in US children, 1979 to 1998. *Neurology* 59: 34–39.

Ganesan V, Hogan A, Shack N, Gordon A *et al* (2000) Outcome after ischaemic stroke in childhood. *Developmental Medicine and Child Neurology* **42**: 455–461.

Ganesan V, Chong W, Cox T, Chawda S (2002) Posterior circulation stroke in childhood: risk factors and recurrence. *Neurology* **59**: 1552–1556.

Ganesan V, Prengler M, McShane M, Wade A, Kirkham F (2003) Investigation of risk factors in children with arterial ischemic stroke. *Annals of Neurology* **53**: 167–173.

Ganesan V, Savvy L, Chong WK, Kirkham FJ (1999) Conventional cerebral angiography in children with ischemic stroke. *Pediatric Neurology* **20**: 38–42.

George BD, Neville BG, Lumley JS (1993) Transcranial revascularisation in childhood and adolescence. *Developmental Medicine and Child Neurology* **35**: 675–682.

Gillick v. *West Norfolk Health Authority* (1985)

Glover J, Mateer C, Yoell C, Speed S (2002) The effectiveness of constraint induced movement therapy in two young children with hemiplegia. *Pediatric Rehabilitation* **5**: 125–131.

Golby AJ, Marks MP, Thompson RC, Steinberg GK *et al* (1999) Direct and combined revascularization in pediatric moyamoya disease. *Neurosurgery* **45**: 50–60.

Goodman R, Yude C (2000) Emotional, behavioural and social consequences. *Congenital hemiplegia. Clinics in Development Medicine* **150**: 166–178.

Gordon AL, Ganesan V, Towell A, Kirkham F (2002) Functional outcome following stroke in children. *Journal of Child Neurology* **17**(6): 429–434.

Hasan I, Wapnick S, Tenner M, Couldwell W (2002) Vertebral artery dissection in children: a comprehensive review. *Pediatric Neurosurgery* **37**: 168–177.

Helps S, Fuggle P, Udwin O, Dick M (2003) Psychosocial and neurocognitive aspects of sickle cell disease. *Child and adolescent mental health* **8**(1): 11–17.

Hogan A, Kirkham F, Isaacs E (2000) Intelligence after stroke in childhood: review of the literature and suggestions for future research. *Journal of Child Neurology* **15**: 325–332.

Hunter JV (2002) Magnetic resonance imaging in pediatric stroke. *Topics in Magnetic Resonance Imaging* **13**(1): 23–38.

Hur J (1995) Review of research on therapeutic interventions for children with cerebral palsy. *Acta Neurologica Scandinavica* **91**: 423–432.

Husson B, Rodesch G, Lasjaunias P, Tardieu M (2003) Magnetic resonance angiography in childhood arterial brain infarcts: a comparative study with contrast angiography. *Stroke* **33**: 1280–1285.

Intercollegiate Stroke Working Party (2004) *National clinical guidelines for stroke: second edition.* London: Royal College of Physicians.

Intercollegiate Working Party for Stroke (2000, update 2002) *National clinical guidelines for stroke.* London: Royal College of Physicians.

Ishikawa T, Houkin K, Kamiyama H, Abe H (1997) Effects of surgical revascularization on outcome of patients with pediatric moyamoya disease. *Stroke* **28**: 1170–1173.

Ketelaar M, Vermeer A, Hart H, van Petegem-van Beek E, Helders P (1997) Effects of a functional therapy program on motor abilities of children with cerebral palsy. *Physical Therapy* **81**: 1534–1545.

Ketelaar M, Vermeer A, Hart H, van Petegem-van Beek E, Helders P (2001) Effects of a functional therapy program on motor abilities of children with cerebral palsy. *Physical Therapy* **81**: 1534–1545.

Kirkham F, Hewes D, Prengler M, Wade A *et al* (2001) Nocturnal hypoxaemia and central-nervous-system events in sickle-cell disease. *Lancet* **357**: 1656–1659.

Kirkham FJ (1999) Stroke in childhood. *Archives of Disease in Childhood* **81**: 85–89.

Kral MC, Brown RT, Hynd GW (2001) Neuropsychological aspects of pediatric sickle cell disease. *Neuropsychology Review* **11**: 179–196.

Kucinski T, Vaterlein O, Glauche V, Fiehler J *et al* (2002) Correlation of apparent diffusion coefficient and computed tomography density in acute ischemic stroke. *Stroke* **33**: 1786–1791.

Lansberg M, Albers G, Beaulieu C, Marks M (2000) Comparison of diffusion-weighted MRI and CT in acute stroke. *Neurology* **54**: 1557–1561.

Lanthier S, Carmant L, David M *et al* (2000) Stroke in children: the coexistence of multiple risk factors predicts poor outcome. *Neurology* **54**: 371–378.

Law M, Cadman D, Rosenbaum P, Walter S *et al* (1991) Neurodevelopmental therapy and upper-extremity inhibitive casting for children with cerebral palsy. *Developmental Medicine and Child Neurology* **33**: 379–387.

Law M, Russell D, Pollock N, Rosenbaum P *et al* (1997) A comparison of intensive neurodevelopmental therapy plus casting and a regular occupational therapy program for children with cerebral palsy. *Developmental Medicine and Child Neurology* **39**: 664–670.

Lees J (1997) Long-term effects of acquired aphasias in childhood. *Paediatric Rehabilitation* **1**: 45–49.

Lees JA, Neville BGR (1990) Acquired aphasia in childhood: case studies of five children. *Aphasiology* **4(5)**: 463–478.

Levy C, Laissy J, Raveau V, Amarenco P (1994) Carotid and vertebral artery dissections: three-dimensional time-of-flight MR angiography and MR imaging versus conventional angiography. *Radiology* **190**: 97–103.

Manco Johnson *et al* (2002) Laboratory testing for thrombophilia in pediatric patients. *Thrombosis and Haemostasis* **88**: 155–156

Matsushima T, Inoue T, Suzuki S, Fujii K (1992) Surgical treatment of moyamoya disease in pediatric patients – comparison between the results of indirect and direct revascularization procedures. *Neurosurgery* **31**: 401–405.

Max JE, Mathews K, Lansing AE, Robertson-Brigitte AM *et al* (2002) Psychiatric disorders after childhood stroke. *Journal of the American Academy of Child & Adolescent Psychiatry* **41**: 555–562.

Morgan AT, Ward EC, Murdoch BE, Kennedy B, Murison R (2003) Incidence, characteristics and predictive factors for dysphagia following pediatric traumatic brain injury. *Journal of Head Trauma Rehabilitation* **18(3)**: 239–251

Mukherjee S, Beresford B, Sloper P (1999) *Unlocking key working: an analysis and evaluation of key worker services for families with disabled children.* Bristol: The Policy Press.

National Association of Paediatric Occupational Therapists (NAPOT) (2000) *Guidelines for good practice.* London: College of Occupational Therapy.

National Institute for Clinical Excellence (2002) *Working together to prevent pressure ulcers: a guide for patients and their carers.* London: National Institute for Clinical Excellence. (**www.nice. org.uk/pdf/clinicalguidelinespressuresorespatleafletenglish.pdf**).

National Institute for Clinical Excellence (2003) Pressure relieving devices: the use of pressure relieving devices for the prevention of pressure ulcers in primary and secondary care. London: NICE. (**www.nice.org.uk**)

Nowak-Gottl U, Strater R, Heinecke A, Junker R *et al* (1999) Lipoprotein (a) and genetic polymorphisms of clotting factor V, prothrombin, and methylenetetrahydrofolate reductase are risk factors of spontaneous ischemic stroke in childhood. *Blood* **94**: 3678–3682.

Nowak-Gottl U, Straeter R, Sebire G, Kirkham FJ (2003) Antithrombotic drug treatment of pediatric patients with ischemic stroke. *Paediatric Drugs* **5(3)**: 167–175.

Olds M, Griebel R, Hoffman H, Craven M *et al* (1987) The surgical treatment of childhood moyamoya disease. *Journal of Neurosurgery* **66**: 675–680.

Ounpuu S, Bell KJ, Davis RB, DeLuca PA (1996) An evaluation of the posterior leaf spring orthosis using joint kinematics and kinetics. *Journal of Pediatric Orthopedics* **16**: 378–384.

Pegelow CH, Adams RJ, McKie V, Abboud M *et al* (1995) Risk of recurrent stroke in patients with sickle cell disease treated with erythrocyte transfusions. *Journal of Pediatrics* **126**: 896–899

Shortland A, Harris C, Gough M, Robinson R (2002) Architecture of the medial gastrocnemius in children with spastic diplegia. *Developmental Medicine and Child Neurology* 44: 158–163.

Stam J, de Bruijn S, DeVeber G (2003) Anticoagulation for cerebral sinus thrombosis (Cochrane Review). In: *The Cochrane Library*, Issue 3, 2003. Chichester, UK: John Wiley and Sons.

Sträter R, Kurnik K, Heller C, Schobess R et al (2001) Aspirin versus low-molecular-weight heparin: antithrombotic therapy in pediatric ischemic stroke patients: a prospective follow-up study. *Stroke* 32: 2554-2558.

Sträter R, Becker S, von Eckardstein A, Heinecke A et al (2002) Prospective assessment of risk factors for recurrent stroke during childhood – a 5-year follow-up study. *Lancet* 360: 1540-1545.

Subcommittee for Perinatal and Pediatric Thrombosis of the Scientific and Standardization Committee of the International Society of Thrombosis and Haemostasis (2002) Laboratory testing for thrombophilia in pediatric patients. *Thrombosis and Haemostasis* 88: 155-156

Sumoza A, de Bisotti R, Sumoza D, Fairbanks V (2002) Hydroxyurea (HU) for prevention of recurrent stroke in sickle cell anemia (SCA). *American Journal of Hematology* 71: 161-165.

Tuffrey C & Pearce A (2003) Transition from paediatric to adult medical services for young people with chronic neurological problems. *Journal of Neurology, Neurosurgery and Psychiatry* 74: 1011-1013.

UNICEF (2003) *Convention on rights of the child.* Geneva: UNICEF.

Van der Weel F, van der Meer A, Lee D (1991) Effect of task on movement control in cerebral palsy: implications for assessment and therapy. *Developmental Medicine and Child Neurology* 33: 419-426.

Vermylen C, Cornu G, Ferster A, Brichard B et al (1998) Haematopoietic stem cell transplantation for sickle cell anaemia: the first 50 patients transplanted in Belgium. *Bone Marrow Transplantation* 22(1): 1-6.

Volman MC, Wijnroks A, Vermeer A (2002) Effect of task on reaching performance in children with spastic hemiparesis. *Clinical Rehabilitation* 16: 684-692.

Walters MC, Storb R, Patience M, Leisenring W et al (2000) Impact of bone marrow transplantation for symptomatic sickle cell disease: an interim report. Multicenter investigation of bone marrow transplantation for sickle cell disease. *Blood* 95(6): 1918-1924.

Wang WC, Kovnar EH, Tonkin IL, Mulhern RK et al (1991) High risk of recurrent stroke after discontinuance of five to twelve years of transfusion therapy in patients with sickle cell disease. *Journal of Pediatrics* 118(3): 377-82.

Ware RE, Zimmerman SA, Schultz WH (1999) Hydroxyurea as an alternative to blood transfusions for the prevention of recurrent stroke in children with sickle cell disease. *Blood* 94: 3022-3026.

Wilimas J, Goff JR, Anderson HR Jr, Langston JW, Thompson E (1980) Efficacy of transfusion therapy for one to two years in patients with sickle cell disease and cerebrovascular accidents. *Journal of Pediatrics* 96(2): 205-208.

Willis JK, Morello A, Davie A, Rice JC, Bennett JT (2002) Forced use treatment of childhood hemiparesis. *Pediatrics* 110: 94-96.

World Health Organization (1978) *Cerebrovascular disorders: a clinical and research classification.* 43. Geneva, WHO.

World Health Organization (2001) *International classification of functioning, disability and health.* Geneva, WHO.

Wraige E, Gordon A, Ganesan V (2003) Behavioural sequelae after arterial ischaemic stroke in childhood. *Developmental Medicine and Child Neurology* 45: 9.

Wright PA & Granat MH (2000) Therapeutic effects of functional electrical stimulation of the upper limb of eight children with cerebral palsy. *Developmental Medicine and Child Neurology* 42: 724-727.

Yasukawa A (1990) Upper extremity casting: adjunct treatment for a child with cerebral palsy hemiplegia. *American Journal of Occupational Therapy* 44: 840-846.

Pegelow CH, Colangelo L, Steinberg M, Wright EC et al (1997) Natural history of blood pressure in sickle cell disease: risks for stroke and death associated with relative hypertension in sickle cell anemia. *American Journal of Medicine* **102**: 171–177.

Pierce SR, Daly K, Gallagher KG, Gershkoff AM, Schaumburg SW (2002) Constraint-induced therapy for a child with hemiplegic cerebral palsy: a case report. *Archives of Physical Medicine and Rehabilitation* **83**: 1462–1463.

Portnoy BA, Herion JC (1972) Neurological manifestations in sickle-cell disease, with a review of the literature and emphasis on the prevalence of hemiplegia. *Annals of Internal Medicine* **76**(4): 643–645.

Powars D, Wilson B, Imbus C, Pegelow C, Allen J (1978) The natural history of stroke in sickle cell disease. *American Journal of Medicine* **65**: 461–471.

Powars D (2000) Management of cerebral vasculopathy in children with sickle cell anaemia. *British Journal of Haematology* **108**: 666–678.

Rana S, Houston PE, Surana N, Shalaby-Rana EI, Castro OL (1997) Discontinuation of long-term transfusion therapy in patients with sickle cell disease and stroke. *Journal of Pediatrics* **131**(5): 757–760.

Reddihough D, King J, Coleman G, Fosang A et al (2002) Functional outcome of botulinum toxin A injections to the lower limbs in cerebral palsy. *Developmental Medicine and Child Neurology* **44**: 820–827.

Romkes J, Brunner R (2002) Comparison of a dynamic and a hinged ankle-foot orthosis by gait analysis in patients with hemiplegic cerebral palsy. *Gait Posture* **15**: 18–24.

Ross S, Engsberg J (2002) Relation between spasticity and strength in individuals with spastic diplegic cerebral palsy. *Developmental Medicine and Child Neurology* **44**: 148–157.

Royal College of Nursing (1999) *The guide to the handling of patients: fourth edition.* London: RCN.

Royal College of Nursing (2001) *Clinical practice guidelines: the recognition and assessment of acute pain in children.* London: RCN. **www.rcn.org.uk/resources/guidelines.php**

Royal College of Nursing (2002) NICE guideline on pressure ulcer risk management and prevention (Guideline B). **www.nice.org.uk/pdf/clinicalguidelinepressureguidancenice.pdf** NICE/RCN.

Royal College of Paediatrics and Child Health and the Neonatal and Pediatric Pharmacists Group (2003) *Medicines for children.* Poole, Dorset: Direct Books.

Royal College of Paediatrics and Child Health (1999) British Association for Community Child Health Child Development and Disability Group: standards for child development services. London: RCPCH.

Royal College of Speech & Language Therapists (2001) *Communicating quality (2).* London: RCSLT.

Royal College of Speech & Language Therapists (2004) *Clinical guideline for disorders of feeding, eating, drinking and swallowing (dysphagia).* London: RCSLT.

Royal College of Speech & Language Therapists (2004) *Core clinical guideline.* London: RCSLT.

Royal College of Speech & Language Therapists (2004) *Clinical guideline for dysarthria.* London: RCSLT.

Rushforth H (1999) Practitioner review: communicating with hospitalised children: review and application of research pertaining to children's understanding of health and illness. *Journal of Child Psychology and Psychiatry and Allied Disciplines* **40**: 683–691.

Russell MO, Goldberg HI, Hodson A, Kim HC et al (1984) Effect of transfusion therapy on arteriographic abnormalities and on recurrence of stroke in sickle cell disease. *Blood* **63**(1): 162–9.

Scothorn D, Price C, Schwartz D, Terrill C et al (2002) Risk of recurrent stroke in children with sickle cell disease receiving blood transfusion therapy for at least five years after initial stroke. *Journal of Paediatrics* **140**: 348–354.

Scottish Intercollegiate Guidelines Network (SIGN) (2001) *SIGN 50: a guideline developer's handbook.* SIGN: Edinburgh.